Update on Ruminant Ultrasound

Editor

SÉBASTIEN BUCZINSKI

VETERINARY CLINICS OF NORTH AMERICA: FOOD ANIMAL PRACTICE

www.vetfood.theclinics.com

Consulting Editor
ROBERT A. SMITH

March 2016 • Volume 32 • Number 1

ELSEVIER

1600 John F. Kennedy Boulevard • Suite 1800 • Philadelphia, Pennsylvania, 19103-2899

http://www.vetfood.theclinics.com

VETERINARY CLINICS OF NORTH AMERICA: FOOD ANIMAL PRACTICE Volume 32, Number 1
March 2016 ISSN 0749-0720, ISBN-13: 978-0-323-323-41669-6

Editor: Patrick Manley
Developmental Editor: Meredith Clinton

Veterinary Clinics of North America: Food Animal Practice (ISSN 0749-0720) is published in March, July, and November by Elsevier Inc., 360 Park Avenue South, New York, NY 10010-1710. Subscription prices are $240.00 per year (domestic individuals), $361.00 per year (domestic institutions), $100.00 per year (domestic students/residents), $265.00 per year (Canadian individuals), $476.00 per year (Canadian institutions), $335.00 per year (international individuals), $476.00 per year (international institutions), and $165.00 per year (international and Canadian students/residents). To receive student/resident rate, orders must be accompanied by name of affiliated institution, date of term, and the signature of program/residency coordinator on institution letterhead. *Clinics* subscription prices. All prices are subject to change without notice. **POSTMASTER:** Send address changes to *Veterinary Clinics of North America: Food Animal Practice*, Elsevier Health Sciences Division, Subscription Customer Service, 3251 Riverport Lane, Maryland Heights, MO 63043. Customer Service (orders, claims, online, change of address): Elsevier Health Sciences Division, Subscription **Customer Service, 3251 Riverport Lane, Maryland Heights, MO 63043. Tel: 1-800-654-2452 (U.S. and Canada);** 314-447-8871 **(ouside U.S. and Canada). Fax: 314-447-8029. E-mail: journalscustomerservice-usa@elsevier.com (for print support); journalsonlinesupport-usa@elsevier.com (for online support).**

Reprints. For copies of 100 or more, of articles in this publication, please contact the Commercial Reprints Department, Elsevier Inc., 360 Park Avenue South, New York, NY 10010-1710. Tel.: 212-633-3874; Fax: 212-633-3820; E-mail: reprints@elsevier.com.

Veterinary Clinics of North America: Food Animal Practice is covered in *Current Contents/Agriculture, Biology and Environmental Sciences, MEDLINE/PubMed (Index Medicus), and Excerpta Medica.*

Contributors

CONSULTING EDITOR

ROBERT A. SMITH, DVM, MS
Diplomate, American Board of Veterinary Practitioners; Veterinary Research and Consulting Services, LLC, Greeley, Colorado

EDITOR

SÉBASTIEN BUCZINSKI, DrVét, DÉS, MSc
Diplomate, American College of Veterinary Internal Medicine; Associate Professor, Department of Clinical Sciences, Faculty of Veterinary Medicine, University of Montreal, Saint-Hyacinthe, Québec, Canada

AUTHORS

JEANNETTE ATTIGER, Med Vet
Department of Farm Animals, University of Zurich, Zurich, Switzerland

MARIE BABKINE, DVM, MSc
Department of Clinical Sciences, Faculté de Médecine Vétérinaire, Université de Montréal, Saint-Hyacinthe, Québec, Canada

JAVIER BLANCO, Dr Med Vet
Department of Animal Medicine and Surgery, Veterinary Faculty, Complutense University of Madrid, Madrid, Spain

HEINRICH BOLLWEIN, PhD, DVM
Diplomate, European College of Bovine Health Management; Professor, Clinic of Reproductive Medicine, Vetsuisse Faculty, University of Zurich, Zurich, Switzerland

UELI BRAUN, Prof Dr Med Vet, Dr Med Vet H C
Diplomate, European College of Bovine Health Management; Professor for Internal Medicine of Cattle, Department of Farm Animals, University of Zurich, Zurich, Switzerland

SÉBASTIEN BUCZINSKI, DrVét, DÉS, MSc
Diplomate, American College of Veterinary Internal Medicine; Associate Professor, Department of Clinical Sciences, Faculté de Médecine Vétérinaire, Université de Montréal, Saint-Hyacinthe, Québec, Canada

PAULO D. CARVALHO, MS
Department of Dairy Science, University of Wisconsin-Madison, Madison, Wisconsin

DAVID FRANCOZ, DVM, MSc
Department of Clinical Sciences, Faculté de Médecine Vétérinaire, Université de Montréal, Saint-Hyacinthe, Québec, Canada

PAUL M. FRICKE, PhD
Department of Dairy Science, University of Wisconsin-Madison, Madison, Wisconsin

IGNACIO A. GÓMEZ DE SEGURA, Dr Med Vet
Diplomate, European College of Veterinary Anaesthesia and Analgesia; Diplomate, European College of Laboratory Animal Medicine; Department of Animal Medicine and Surgery, Veterinary Faculty, Complutense University of Madrid, Madrid, Spain

JULIO O. GIORDANO, PhD
Department of Animal Science, Cornell University, Ithaca, New York

VÉRONIQUE BERNIER GOSSELIN, DVM, MSc
Department of Veterinary Medicine and Surgery, College of Veterinary Medicine, University of Missouri, Columbia, Missouri

MAIKE HEPPELMANN, DVM
Clinic for Cattle, University of Veterinary Medicine Hannover, Hannover, Germany

JOHANNES LÜTTGENAU, DVM
Clinic of Reproductive Medicine, Vetsuisse-Faculty, University of Zurich, Zurich, Switzerland

KATHARYN JEAN MITCHELL, BVSc, DVCS
Diplomate, American College of Veterinary Internal Medicine; Clinic for Equine Internal Medicine, Vetsuisse Faculty, University of Zurich, Zurich, Switzerland

ANNETTE M. O'CONNOR, MVSc, DVSc, FANZCVs
Department of Veterinary Diagnostic and Production Animal Medicine, College of Veterinary Medicine, Iowa State University, Ames, Iowa

THERESA L. OLLIVETT, DVM, PhD
Diplomate, American College of Veterinary Internal Medicine; Department of Medical Sciences, University of Wisconsin-Madison, School of Veterinary Medicine, Madison, Wisconsin

MICHELA RE, Dr Med Vet
Department of Animal Medicine and Surgery, Veterinary Faculty, Complutense University of Madrid, Madrid, Spain

ALESSANDRO RICCI, DVM
Department of Veterinary Science, University of Torino, Grugliasco, Italy

COLIN CLAUDIO SCHWARZWALD, Prof Dr Med Vet, PhD
Diplomate, American College of Veterinary Internal Medicine; Diplomate, European College of Equine Internal Medicine; Clinic for Equine Internal Medicine, Vetsuisse Faculty, University of Zurich, Zurich, Switzerland

PHIL SCOTT, BVM&S, DVM&S, MPhil, DSHP, FHEA, FRCVS
Reader, Diplomate, European College of Bovine Health Management; Diplomate, European College of Small Ruminant Health Management; Division of Veterinary Clinical Sciences, R(D)SVS, University of Edinburgh, Easter Bush, Midlothian, United Kingdom

RICHARD GREGORY TAIT Jr, MS, PhD, PAS (Professional Animal Scientist)
Research Geneticist, Genetics, Breeding, and Animal Health Research Unit, USDA, ARS, US Meat Animal Research Center, Clay Center, Nebraska

Contents

Ultrasonography is used by bovine practitioners more for reproductive
issues rather than as a diagnostic test for medical and surgical diseases.
This article reviews the specific challenges and standards concerning
the reporting of studies on diagnostic accuracy of ultrasound in cattle for
non-reproductive issues. Specific biases and applicability concerns in
studies reporting ultrasonography as a diagnostic test are also reviewed.
Better understanding of these challenges will help the practitioner to interpret and apply diagnostic accuracy study results depending on the field
context. Examples of application of sensitivity and specificity results in a
clinical context are given using the Bayes theorem.

Thoracic ultrasonography (TUS) in young cattle has recently gained
momentum as an accurate and practical tool for identifying the lung lesions associated with bovine respiratory disease. As cattle producers
increasingly seek input from their veterinarians on respiratory health
issues, bovine practitioners should consider adding TUS to their practice
models. This article discusses the relevant literature regarding TUS in
young cattle, current acceptable techniques, and practical on-farm
applications.

 Videos showing echocardiographic examples of congenital heart
defects in calves accompany this article

Congenital heart disease should be considered when evaluating calves
with chronic respiratory signs, failure to thrive, poor growth, or if a murmur
is heard on physical examination. Echocardiography is currently the gold
standard for diagnosing congenital heart defects. A wide variety of
defects, either alone or in combination with a ventricular septal defect,
are possible. A standardized approach using sequential segmental
analysis is required to fully appreciate the nature and severity of more
complex malformations. The prognosis for survival varies from guarded

to poor and depends on the hemodynamic relevance of the defects and the degree of cardiac compensation.

Ultrasonography enables the examiner to detect very small amounts of fluid in the peritoneal cavity and to determine its location, amount, and sonographic features. The pathologic process responsible for the ascites, for example, ileus, hepatic fibrosis, thrombosis of the caudal vena cava, or traumatic reticuloperitonitis, can often be identified. Abdominocentesis and analysis of the aspirated fluid allow differentiation of inflammatory and non-inflammatory ascites, as well as the diagnosis of uroperitoneum, hemoperitoneum, chylous ascites, and bile peritonitis.

This article describes the ultrasonographic findings of the reticulum, rumen, omasum, abomasum, and liver of calves from birth to 100 days of age. Reticular motility is used to exemplify how the forestomach function in calves progresses and gradually approaches that of adult cattle. The ultrasonographic examination of the esophageal groove reflex and the investigation of factors affecting esophageal groove closure are described. The ultrasonographic findings of the forestomachs and abomasum of calves with ruminal drinker syndrome are discussed. The article concludes with the description of the ultrasonographic examination of the liver.

Ultrasonography is useful for the visualization of the spinal cord and associated structures, and facilitates the safe collection of cerebrospinal fluid from the atlanto-occipital space in cattle. This technique is less stressful than the blind puncture technique because it does not require strong ventroflexion of the head. Furthermore, painful puncture of the spinal cord can largely be avoided when ultrasound guidance is used.

Diseases of the middle ear or the larynx are not frequent in cattle, but their diagnosis can be challenging for veterinary practitioners in the field. This article presents the ultrasonography of these two anatomic structures in order to provide new diagnostic tools to veterinary practitioners in the field. Brief anatomic reminders are first reported. Then, the scanning techniques and normal images are described. Finally, abnormal images of specific conditions are presented.

Superficial nerves can be visualized through ultrasonography in the cattle and facilitate local anesthetic disposition around nerve structures. Expected advantages include a higher successful rate of nerve block improving the degree and duration of the block. Among others, conduction nerves of clinical interest in cattle include the paravertebral nerves, nerves of the epidural space, the brachial plexus, and the sciatic and femoral nerves, and nerves of the head.

Transrectal color Doppler ultrasonography is a useful technique to get new information about physiologic and pathophysiologic alterations of the uterus and ovaries in female cattle. During all reproductive stages characteristic changes in uterine blood flow are observed. Cows with puerperal disturbances show delayed decrease in uterine blood flow in the first few weeks postparturition compared with healthy cows. Measurement of follicular blood flow is used to identify normally developing follicles and predict superovulatory response. Determination of luteal blood is more reliable than B-mode sonography to distinguish between functional and nonfunctional corpora lutea. Color Doppler ultrasonography is a promising tool to improve reproductive management in female cattle.

The first part of this article defines the attributes of the ideal pregnancy test and describes the direct and indirect methods for pregnancy diagnosis in dairy cows that are currently available, and that have the potential to replace transrectal palpation. Second, this new technology must be practically integrated into a systematic on-farm reproductive management strategy and empirically demonstrated to exceed the status quo of the industry in reproductive performance. Finally, a future direction for research and technology in the area of early pregnancy diagnosis in dairy cows is presented, and the overall conclusions of the ideas presented herein are drawn.

 Videos of ultrasound examples accompany this article

Modern portable ultrasound scan machines provide the veterinary clinician with an inexpensive and noninvasive method to further examine sheep on farms, which should take no more than 5 minutes with the results available immediately. Repeat examinations allow monitoring of the disease process and assessment of therapy. 5 MHz linear array scanners can be used for most organs except the heart and right kidney. Transthoracic ultrasonography is particularly useful for critical evaluation of lung and

VETERINARY CLINICS OF NORTH AMERICA: FOOD ANIMAL PRACTICE

THE CLINICS ARE NOW AVAILABLE ONLINE!
Access your subscription at:
www.theclinics.com

VETERINARY CLINICS OF NORTH AMERICA FOOD ANIMAL PRACTICE

FORTHCOMING ISSUES

July 2016
Bovine Theriogenology
Robert L. Larson, Editor

November 2016
Bovine Surgery
David Anderson and Andrew Niehaus, Editors

March 2017
Food Animal Neurology
Kevin Washburn, Editor

RECENT ISSUES

November 2015
Feedlot Production Medicine
Daniel U. Thomson and Brad J. White, Editors

July 2015
Feedlot Processing and Arrival Cattle Management
Brad J. White and Daniel U. Thomson, Editors

March 2015
Bovine Clinical Pharmacology
Michael D. Apley, Editor

ISSUE OF RELATED INTEREST

Veterinary Clinics of North America: Equine Practice
August 2015, Vol. 31, No. 2
Equine Pathology and Laboratory Diagnosis
Bruce S. Webster and Colleen P. Leuratti, Editors

THE CLINICS ARE NOW AVAILABLE ONLINE!

Access your subscription at:
www.theclinics.com

Preface

We Need More Studies on the Diagnostic and Prognostic Use of Ultrasound in Ruminants!

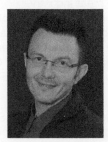

Sébastien Buczinski, Dr Vét, DÉS, MSc
Editor

The first issue of the *Veterinary Clinics of North America: Food Animal Practice* devoted to bovine ultrasonography was published 7 years ago in 2009. Since then, much progress has been made with a wider availability on-farm of high-quality ultrasound units. There are also new publications mentioning exciting new indications for this imaging test. For these reasons, we thought it was a good idea to update the 2009 issue. For this new issue, we insisted on new indications of ultrasound as well as specific applications that were not developed previously. In order to maintain development and use of ultrasound on the farm and to convince farmers of the usefulness of this tool, we need to report studies comparing the accuracy of this test to the current techniques of diagnosis as well as a second step showing the improvement of patient/herd management when using that test. We need more studies showing the impact of ultrasound in the diagnosis and the prognosis of ruminant health conditions (at both individual and herd level) in order to demonstrate the added value of this ancillary test. We therefore included a specific article focusing on the challenges in reporting diagnostic accuracy of ultrasound.

At the individual level, ultrasonography of the spinal cord, peripheral nerve, tympanic bulla, larynx, and congenital heart defects is a new promising application for a better diagnosis, or anesthesia in cattle. We also included a specific article on the ultrasonographic assessment of causes of ascites, which is a problem that the practitioner may face. A specific article on calves' gastrointestinal system has also been added. This article illustrates how ultrasound can be used not only for diagnostic purposes but also as a tool in research to assess gastrointestinal response under experimental conditions. Ultrasonography can also be used for diagnosis of various diseases in small ruminants; a specific article has therefore been added for this application.

Vet Clin Food Anim 32 (2016) xi–xii
http://dx.doi.org/10.1016/j.cvfa.2016.01.017
0749-0720/16/$ – see front matter © 2016 Published by Elsevier Inc.

vetfood.theclinics.com

Concerning the specific use of this imaging technique at the herd level, evaluation of the reproductive tract is still the main reason for ultrasonographic use in cattle, and for this reason, two specific articles on that topic have been added (one on Doppler use and a second that emphasizes the comparative aspects of several tests to assess early pregnancy, including ultrasound). The on-farm assessment of bovine respiratory disease (BRD) -induced lung lesions by thoracic ultrasound to monitor BRD at the individual and herd level has also gained interest. Finally, we have also added a specific article on ultrasonographic assessment for measuring conformation and carcass quality, which is a topic of interest for everyone involved in the meat industry.

I want to sincerely thank all the internationally recognized collaborating authors who accepted to contribute to this issue. Their high quality articles prove that ultrasound has broad applications. I also thank Dr Bob Smith and the Elsevier editorial team for their help during the publication process. I hope that the readers of *Veterinary Clinics of North America: Food Animal Practice* will enjoy this new issue with multiple online supplements!

Sébastien Buczinski, Dr Vét, DÉS, MSc
Department of Clinical Sciences
Faculté de Médecine Vétérinaire
Université de Montréal
CP 5000
Saint-Hyacinthe, Québec, Canada J2S 7C6

E-mail address:
s.buczinski@umontreal.ca

Specific Challenges in Conducting and Reporting Studies on the Diagnostic Accuracy of Ultrasonography in Bovine Medicine

Sébastien Buczinski, DrVét, DES, MSc[a],*,
Annette M. O'Connor, MVSc, DVSc, FANZCVs[b]

KEYWORDS

- Imaging • Bias • Sensitivity • Specificity

KEY POINTS

- Studies reporting diagnostic accuracy of ultrasound for medical and surgical diseases of cattle need to be consistently reported in order to improve their applicability in private practice.
- Specific challenges need to be addressed when designing studies on ultrasound diagnostic accuracy to avoid any bias that could affect the reported accuracy (in terms of sensitivity and specificity).
- Improving the reporting of the studies and trying to avoid any bias would help with faster dissemination of ultrasonography as an effective diagnostic test in bovine medicine and surgery.

INTRODUCTION

Bovine ultrasonography has gained popularity since the early 1980s, first as a tool for assessing the reproductive tract. The medical and surgical indications of ultrasonography developed in parallel with its use as an interesting noninvasive tool in humans and in veterinary species. The portability of ultrasonography, as well as its relatively low cost, are factors associated with its more general use as a diagnostic test by bovine practitioners for reproductive management of cattle. The use of ultrasonography for nonreproductive purposes has also gained popularity, however, this use is far less common than reproductive applications.[1]

Disclosure: The authors have nothing to disclose.
[a] Department of Clinical Sciences, Faculté de médecine vétérinaire, Université de Montréal, St-Hyacinthe, Québec CP 5000, Canada; [b] Department of Veterinary Diagnostic and Production Animal Medicine, College of Veterinary Medicine, Iowa State University, IA 50010, USA
* Corresponding author.
E-mail address: s.buczinski@umontreal.ca

As with any diagnostic test used in the medical and surgical decision process, the validity and usefulness of ultrasonography for detection of disease first needs to be judged in comparison with other testing options. Comparisons are made between the test of interest, referred to as the index test, and a gold standard test or reference standard test. Technically, the gold standard test is 100% accurate. An imperfect reference standard may also be used for comparison when a gold standard is unavailable or not feasible. For example, pneumonia could be diagnosed in a study using a reference standard, such as the presence of fever AND nasal discharge AND cough AND dyspnea (a definition that may be specific but lacks sensitivity), but the gold standard examination would be necropsy and isolation of pathogens which cannot be performed routinely because of obvious side effects.

Comparative diagnostic test studies with binomial (2 levels) categorical outcomes, such as diseased and nondiseased, summarize the characteristics of an index test using sensitivity (Se, number of patients who had an index test positive and are gold standard test positive ÷ number of patients who are gold standard test positive expressed as a proportion or percentage) and specificity (Sp, number of patients who had an index test negative and gold standard test negative ÷ number of patients who are gold standard test negative) (**Table 1**). If an imperfect reference standard is used, then the relative sensitivity (index test positive and reference standard positive ÷ test positive based on imperfect reference standard) and relative specificity (index test negative and reference standard negative ÷ negative based on imperfect reference standard) can be calculated. Many investigators do not distinguish between true and relative summary measures. However, designing studies to accurately measure sensitivity and specificity requires careful planning. Apart from random error, sources of systematic bias can create biased measures of Se and Sp; as a consequence, it is important that practitioners understand these systematic biases.

The objective of this article is to review the specific challenges and standards for reporting diagnostic (STARD) accuracy studies, and the methodological issues that can introduce bias into studies reporting ultrasonography as a diagnostic test in bovine medical and surgical disorders. As an outline of the article, the following topics are covered:

- Phases of testing assessment and study designs
- Reporting guidelines for diagnostic test assessment studies relating to imaging

Table 1
Determination of accuracy of the parameters of ultrasonography (index test) compared with a reference standard test that may or may not be a gold standard test

	Reference Standard +	Reference Standard −	
Ultrasonography +	TP	FP	TP + FP
Ultrasonography −	FN	TN	FN + TN
	TP + FN	FP + TN	n

TP + FN = positive cases (reference standard positive cases); TN + FP = negative cases (reference standard negative cases); TP + FP = cases that were ultrasonography positive; FN + TN = cases that were ultrasonography negative; n = total number of cases included in the study. Accuracy measurement: Se = TP/(TP + FN); Sp = TN/(TN + FP); these accuracy measures (sensitivity and specificity) are relative sensitivity and relative specificity if the reference standard used is not 100% accurate; PPV = TP/(TP + FP); NPV = TN/(TN + FN); PLR = Se/(1 − Sp); NLR = (1 − Se)/Sp; DOR = PLR/NLR = TP × TN/(FP × FN) = (Se × Sp)/((1 − Se) × (1 − Sp)).

Abbreviations: DOR, diagnostic odds ratio; FN, false-negative cases; FP, false-positive cases; NLR, negative likelihood ratio; PLR, positive likelihood ratio; TN, true-negative cases; TP, true-positive cases.

- Sources of error in diagnostic test assessment studies relating to imaging
- Practical examples using results of ultrasound accuracy study in daily bovine practice

PHASES OF TESTING ASSESSMENT AND STUDY DESIGNS

Interventions do not suddenly become candidates for clinical trials; there is a process of establishing likely efficacy before conducting clinical trials. Pilot studies without control groups, followed by small phase 1 studies or animal experiments provide evidence for the conduct of clinical trials of interventions. The same can be said for diagnostic tests.[2] Initially, small feasibility studies are conducted to identify if the diagnostic method has potential. For example, a study was performed to compare the acoustic characteristics of normal bovine liver with those of liver with abscesses showing that ultrasonography has the potential to differentiate these situations.[3] These types of hypotheses-generating studies are frequently case series mentioning ultrasonographic findings in cattle with a specific disease. An ultrasonographic study in 11 cows describing liver ultrasound characteristics, where abscessation was confirmed by centesis or necropsy, was also reported.[4]

Providing the test shows promise, it should then go forward to the next phase of validation and be compared with other testing options (such a study is comparative and is sometimes called a diagnostic test assessment study (DTA)). This article is mainly concerned with this phase of testing, because it is most common in the imaging literature. Comparative studies have the diagnostic test characteristics (Se, Sp, and likelihood ratio [LR]) (see **Table 1**) as the outcome. Other outcomes that researchers might report from DTA studies include positive predictive value, negative predictive value, or accuracy. However, as these later outcomes are affected by prevalence, they are not generalizable. Ultrasonography has also been used for diagnosing liver abscesses in beef calves and compared with slaughterhouse results and blood liver enzyme activity.[5]

Having shown that the tests are accurate by some measure of interest, the next phase of diagnostic test development might be a study of clinical value. Such studies try to determine the true clinical value of the test, rather than its diagnostic test characteristics, that is, how much patient outcomes change with the incorporation of the assay into clinical care compared with an alternative or none. Studies of this nature measure a comparative effect size, such as risk ratio, hazard ratio, or a mean difference of an outcome of clinical importance rather than diagnostic test characteristics. This phase of diagnostic testing assessment is rare in humans and even rarer in animals. Patients are randomized to receive 1 of several testing protocols and followed over time to see different outcomes. Such designs are very similar to clinical trials for treatment interventions; however, such designs have complex ethical implications and are rarely conducted. Finally, pragmatic before-and-after studies can compare outcomes before and after the adoption of a new assay into general practice. Such studies are often biased because of confounding (eg, the index test was not the only difference in case management but change of standard care during the study period could also lead to different results) and are not discussed here.

Two general designs exist for DTA studies. Unfortunately, unlike observational studies or trials, the terminology of DTA studies is somewhat fluid but general designs are considered either 1-gate designs/cohort designs or 2-gate/case-control designs (**Fig. 1**).[6] The use of the terms cohort or case-control can be somewhat confusing for people more familiar with these terms in observational studies, where cohort would

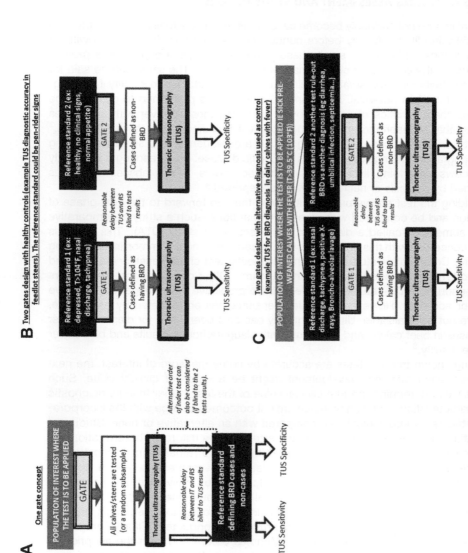

Fig. 1. One-gate (cohort) and 2-gate (case-control) designs used in diagnostic test accuracy study. The 1-gate (A) design is applied when the whole population (or a random sample) is tested with the same reference standard (gate) and index test. The 2-gate design is noted when different reference standards are applied for defining diseased (gate 1) and nondiseased (gate 2) animals. The nondiseased animals could either be healthy control animals (B) or animals with an alternative diagnosis than the disease under study (C). The 2-gate design (especially in the case of healthy controls) frequently overestimates diagnostic accuracy.

often imply a longitudinal component. Here, instead, the term cohort simply refers to a single group.

The 1-gate/cohort design is usually preferred for DTA. For the 1-gate design all included patients go through a single "gate" (eg, clinical signs or a population of interest) and then are cross-classified according to both assays, that is, ultrasonographic and reference standard results. Because there is no previous difference in the selection of affected and nonaffected cases using different "gates," this type of design is less prone to bias for test accuracy determination when compared with the 2-gate (case-control) approach.[7] The 2-gate approach differs from the 1-gate design because 2 populations (disease-positive [cases] and disease-negative [controls] patients) are selected using different approaches. The goal is that this approach would provide the same comparison as the 1-gate design; however, in reality as the cases and controls are often defined by different inclusion criteria or testing protocols, the risk of systematic bias is higher (see **Fig. 1**B, C).

REPORTING GUIDELINES FOR DIAGNOSTIC TEST ASSESSMENT STUDIES AS THEY RELATE TO IMAGING

As with any primary research study, the description of the method should be comprehensive enough to enable replication. Comprehensive reporting is also critical for enabling the assessment of biases that will occur in a second step. For diagnostic test accuracy studies in cattle, it is therefore of primary importance to generate good quality data (high internal validity) that could be used in the intended setting of application, and to give practitioners confidence to use ultrasonography in their practical setting. The aim of comprehensive reporting should be that the readers assess the potential for bias (internal validity), assess external validity, and obtain common accuracy parameters such as Se and Sp, prevalence of disease, and the diagnostic odds ratio (DOR), which is a global indicator of general accuracy (see **Table 1**).

To improve reporting of diagnostic accuracy studies, the STARD accuracy studies have been developed in human medical research.[8] In the absence of specific recommendations for animal studies, these reporting recommendations can be considered as practical guidelines that could be applied in veterinary medicine.[8,9] The STARD checklist consists of 25 items that should be included in any report of comparative diagnostic test studies. The STARD checklist (**Table 2**) is not specific for ultrasonography studies so we have attempted to provide specific details that should be included for ultrasonography studies in bovine medical issues (see **Table 2**). We strongly encourage future studies on diagnostic accuracy of ultrasonography in bovine medical and surgical diseases to follow the STARD guidelines because they can be used to standardize the reports, and may also be helpful for performing future systematic reviews on diagnostic tests such as ultrasonography.

STARD item 8 includes specific information about the index test (ultrasonography) and should be thoroughly explained. This includes information about the machine, including the probe size, model, manufacturer, and software version. The specifics of the probe settings used include frequency (MHz), depth of examination (cm), focus, gain, and the approach to handling animals, including any restraints or sedation required.

For STARD item 13, the intraoperator and interoperator repeatability should also be included as potential confounding variables of test accuracy.[10,11] The operator's level of expertise should also be reported because it may have an effect on the accuracy of the test.[12] For example, cardiac ultrasonography studies are often performed by people with a strong background in echocardiography in a hospital setting, and therefore

Table 2
Standard for the reporting of diagnostic accuracy studies checklist according to Bossuyt and colleagues[8] and specific information adapted for studies on diagnostic ultrasonography in cattle

Section and Topic	Item	Description of the Item (STARD)[a]	Specific Information for Ultrasound Studies in Cattle[b]	On Page
Title/Abstract/Keywords	1	Identify the article as a study of diagnostic accuracy (recommend MeSH heading "sensitivity and specificity")	Include ultrasound and accuracy terms	—
Introduction	2	State the research questions or study aims, such as estimating diagnostic accuracy or comparing accuracy between tests or across participant groups	Rationale of the study indicating why ultrasonographic diagnosis is required	—
Methods				
Participants	3	Describe the study population: the inclusion and exclusion criteria, setting, and locations where the data were collected	Cows, calves, beef, dairy, male, female? Any farm clustering?	—
	4	Describe patient recruitment: was recruitment based on presenting symptoms, results from previous tests, or the fact that the participants had received the (evaluated) index tests or the (golden) reference standard?	Recruitment based on ultrasonographic results or the gold standard test?	—
	5	Describe patient sampling: was the study population a consecutive series of participants defined by the selection criteria in items 3 and 4? If not, specify how participants were further selected	—	—
	6	Describe data collection: was data collection planned before the index test and reference standard were performed (prospective study) or after (retrospective study)?	—	—
Test methods	7	Describe the reference standard and its rationale	—	—
	8	Describe the technical specifications of the materials and methods involved including how and when measurements were taken, and/or cite references for index tests and reference standard	Specify the ultrasound unit used, the probe required, and any specific setting needed	—
	9	Describe definition of and rationale for the units, cut-offs, and/or categories of the results of the index tests and the reference standard	Specify criteria used to define a positive/negative ultrasonography examination as well as any doubtful category	—
	10	Describe the number, training, and expertise of the persons executing and reading the index tests and the reference standard	Briefly describe the operator's previous knowledge with bovine ultrasound	—
	11	Describe whether or not the readers of the index tests and reference standard were blind (masked) to the results of the other test and describe any other clinical information available to the readers	Interpretation of ultrasonographic images/loop made cow-side or offline?	—

Statistical methods	12	Describe methods for calculating or comparing measures of diagnostic accuracy, and the statistical methods used to quantify uncertainty (eg, 95% confidence intervals)	—	—
	13	Describe methods for calculating test reproducibility, if done	—	—
Results				
Participants	14	Report when study was done, including beginning and ending dates of recruitment	—	—
	15	Report clinical and demographic characteristics of the study population (eg, age, sex, spectrum of presenting symptoms, comorbidity, current treatments, recruitment centers)	Beef vs dairy, calves or adults, hospital vs field setting	—
	16	Report the number of participants satisfying the criteria for inclusion who did or did not undergo the index tests and/or the reference standard; describe why participants failed to receive either test (a flow diagram is strongly recommended)	Any limitation of the ultrasonographic examination because of cattle characteristics (body condition score or temperament) should be included	—
Test results	17	Report time interval from the index tests to the reference standard, and any treatment administered between	If necropsy is used as a gold standard, the delay between ultrasonography and necropsy should be reported	—
	18	Report distribution of severity of disease (define criteria) in those with the target condition; other diagnoses in participants without the target condition	—	—
	19	Report a cross-tabulation of the results of the index tests (including indeterminate and missing results) by the results of the reference standard; for continuous results, the distribution of the test results by the results of the reference standard	—	—
	20	Report any adverse events from performing the index tests or the reference standard	—	—

(continued on next page)

Table 2
(continued)

Section and Topic	Item	Description of the Item (STARD)[a]	Specific Information for Ultrasound Studies in Cattle[b]	On Page
Estimates	21	Report estimates of diagnostic accuracy and measures of statistical uncertainty (eg, 95% confidence intervals)	Sensitivity, specificity, prevalence of the disease, diagnostic odds ratio, likelihood ratio … covariates that could mitigate diagnostic accuracy (eg, body size or condition score that may affect image quality)	—
	22	Report how indeterminate results, missing responses, and outliers of the index tests were handled	Report the number of animals where ultrasonography could not be performed because of a temperament issues or other factor (fat, depth)	—
	23	Report estimates of variability of diagnostic accuracy between subgroups of participants, readers, or hospitals, if done	Is there any variation of accuracy because of age, sex, or any measured covariable?	—
	24	Report estimates of test reproducibility, if done	—	—
Discussion	25	Discuss the clinical applicability of the study findings	—	—

[a] *Reproduced from* the STARD official Web site http://www.stard-statement.org/; with permission.

[b] Specific details added by the authors for ultrasonography accuracy studies.

Adapted from Bossuyt PM, Reitsma JB, Bruns DE, et al. STARD 2015: an updated list of essential items for reporting diagnostic accuracy studies. Available at http://www.stard-statement.org/.

the results may not represent the accuracy that the average bovine practitioner would obtain with the technique when performing cardiac ultrasonography on the farm.

The patient characteristics that potentially influence the quality of the examination and its potential accuracy should be described.[13] It is important that every article report the total number of patients who were initially included and those in whom ultrasonography could not be performed adequately (STARD items 16, 19, and 22). This information will enable the end users to understand the study population and the external population to which the results might relate. As a practical example, if the study reports an assessment of thoracic ultrasonography for the diagnosis of bovine respiratory disease (BRD) on dairy calves (items 15 and 16), it would be reasonable for the end users to consider that the approach might be less sensitive in heavier feedlot calves more than 100 days on feed because of poor penetration of the ultrasounds and heavy forelimb musculature. In this case the reader would be able to see that this test would not be practical if applied during the late feeding period (in calves >454–544 kg [1000–1200 lb]).

The STARD checklist does not allow direct assessment of the quality of the study. The list was initially developed to improve the completeness of study reporting and to try to standardize the diagnostic accuracy of the study content. When trying to assess the quality and validity of an ultrasonography study, other tools should be used that focus on this risk of bias in every study, as well as on specific applicability concerns (ie, can the results of a particular study be used depending on the specific practitioner context?).

VALIDITY AND BIASES IN DIAGNOSTIC TEST ASSESSMENT STUDIES AS THEY RELATE TO IMAGING USING ULTRASONOGRAPHY

Diagnostic test assessment studies have unique issues relating to internal and external validity that differ from studies of interventions. Several tools have been developed to determine the internal and external validity of diagnostic test accuracy. Among these tools, the Quality Assessment of Diagnostic Accuracy Studies-2 (QUADAS-2) is widely used when assessing the potential for bias.[14] The QUADAS-2 tool (Table 3) assesses 4 different areas of study design that relate to internal validity: patient selection, index test (ultrasonography), reference standard (gold standard or pseudo-gold standard that is used to define the disease status), flow, and timing. QUADAS-2 refers to these areas of study design as domains. QUADAS-2 also assesses 3 other domains that relate to external validity or applicability concerns: patient selection, index test, and reference standard. QUADAS-2, although not exhaustive, is a useful approach for assessing studies of diagnostic test accuracy, including imaging techniques such as ultrasonography. QUADAS-2 is included as a quality assessment tool in many systematic reviews of diagnostic test accuracy. The QUADAS-2 results for any domain are referred to as high (risk of bias or applicability concerns), low, or unclear. The unclear result is noted when the information is not reported or reported with insufficient detail to categorize the domain as low or high.

SOURCES OF ERROR IN DIAGNOSTIC TEST ASSESSMENT STUDIES AS THEY RELATE TO IMAGING

As with any form of primary research, diagnostic tests designed to assess the value of ultrasonic imaging are subject to biases. Although rare, trials of the clinical value of ultrasonic imaging can be assessed using the risk of bias tools designed for clinical trials.[15] However, because of the goal, estimation of the accuracy of diagnostic test characteristics studies has different sources of bias. It is critical that readers grasp these sources of bias so that they can determine the potential for bias in the results.

Table 3
Summary of the study characteristics assessed by the Quality Assessment of Diagnostic Accuracy Studies-2 developed by Whiting and colleagues[14]

QUADAS Phases	Items Assessed	Specific Points to Assess in the Reported Study	Rating	No.
Phase 1	Description of study	Stating the review question (setting, intended use of IT, presentation, previous testing)	No	1
		Patients	No	2
		IT	No	3
		RS and TC	No	4
Phase 2	Representation of the flow	Drawing a flow diagram of the study	No	5
Phase 3	—	Risk of bias and applicability	—	—
Patient selection	Risk of bias	Methods of patients selection/consecutive or random sample/case-control/inappropriate exclusions	Low/high/unclear	6
	Concerns regarding applicability	Concerns regarding the fact that included patients do not match the review question	Low/high/unclear	7
Index test	Risk of bias	Description of the test/interpretation blind to reference standard/pre-specified threshold rather than data driven	Low/high/unclear	8
	Concerns regarding applicability	Concerns regarding the fact that IT or its conduct, interpretation do not match the review question	Low/high/unclear	9
Reference test	Risk of bias	Description of the RS, its accuracy, interpretation blind to IT	Low/high/unclear	10
	Concerns regarding applicability	Concerns regarding the fact that the RS or TC differs from the review question	Low/high/unclear	11
Flow and timing	Risk of bias	Interval between IT and RS, same RS for all the patients, inclusion of all patients in the analysis	Low/high/unclear	12

Abbreviations: IT, index test; RS, reference standard; TC, target condition.
Adapted from Whiting PF, Rutjes AW, Westwood ME, et al. QUADAS-2: a revised tool for the quality assessment of diagnostic accuracy studies. Ann Intern Med 2011;155:530.

The ability of end users to assess bias is linked to the comprehensive nature of reporting.[16] There are numerous studies that provide information about biases in diagnostic test accuracy,[14,17] and several that are specific to imaging although not necessarily only ultrasonography.[2,18] Here we provide examples of how such a bias might occur, rather than a detailed description of the bias as already discussed in other articles. The names of the bias might not be always consistent across the articles and we use those listed by QUADAS-2.[14]

INTERNAL VALIDATION OF ULTRASONOGRAPHY IN DIAGNOSTIC STUDIES: SYSTEMATIC ERROR
Biases That May Occur in Imaging Studies as a Result of the Approach to Patient Selection

Spectrum bias
Perhaps the most readily recognizable bias in diagnostic test assessment, spectrum bias, refers to the concept that most tests identify extreme cases and healthy patients, and it is the cases in the middle that present a difficulty.[18,19] If the study population does not represent the full spectrum of cases, then estimates of Se and Sp will likely be biased. The direction of bias associated with spectrum bias is usually overestimation of Se and Sp. The approach to reducing spectrum bias is based in the study design. One-gate studies that select a subset of the source population to be in the study using random selection methods or census of the population, that is, all patients presented consecutively, are least susceptible to spectrum bias. The study design most commonly associated with spectrum bias is the 2-gate/case-control design, which is discouraged for this reason. Two-gate studies may be of interest in the first step of test assessment as a practical way to see the potential of the test, or when the disease to assess is rare but the potential for bias remains. Previously, 1 of the authors compared the ultrasonographic thickness of the cardiac valves in cattle with a confirmed diagnosis of valvular endocarditis (reference standard, necropsy) with healthy cattle from local dairy farms (2-gate with healthy controls; see **Fig. 1B**), and a group of animals with various cardiorespiratory diseases (2-gate with alternative diagnostic group; see **Fig. 1C**).[20] In this study, the extreme case selection with endocarditic cattle that were submitted to necropsy (which may also indicate higher chances of advanced stage of endocarditis and more severe lesions) compared with healthy cows likely overestimated the diagnostic accuracy of ultrasonography.

Continuing with the example of bovine endocarditis and echocardiography, the exclusion of cases with a reasonable suspicion of endocarditis that had never been necropsied would favor overestimation of Se/Sp (ie, some of the non-necropsied cases [maybe less severe symptoms] could be false-positive [ultrasonography positive with no endocarditis] or false-negative [ultrasonography negative with endocarditis], and therefore never tested using the gold standard). Referral hospitals may also have issues with spectrum bias because only difficult or chronic cases are referred, for example, with chronic BRD.[21]

Spectrum bias is usually considered an issue of internal validity associated with overestimation of diagnostic test characteristics. However, spectrum bias might also be recognized as an external validity issue. If the study population comprises only extreme cases such as those presented at a referral hospital, then the estimates of Se and Sp might be considered biased if the end user plans to apply the test to a population with a broad spectrum, or valid if the end user is also in a referral hospital that sees only that spectrum of cases. In endocarditis, the "apparent" Se of cardiac ultrasonography in a hospital study where the reference standard was necropsy (ie, end spectrum of the disease because of referral and the type of reference standard used) could be higher than the "true" Se of cardiac ultrasonography when applied to the whole spectrum of endocarditis cases that may be seen by a bovine practitioner in private practice. In this way, we would propose that external validity and internal validity can overlap somewhat, and hence it is essential that end users assess these issues before application of the data.

Biases That May Occur in Imaging Studies as a Result of the Approach to Conducting the Index Test or Reference Text

The term "index test" in DTA studies refers to the test being evaluated, which in this article refers to ultrasonography. The reference test is that which is being used as a comparison (ideally a gold standard or the current diagnostic test). The following sources of bias do not relate to the study population but the execution of the assay.

Diagnostic review bias and incorporation bias

This bias relates to the absence of blinding of the reference tests result when the index test is carried out. Knowledge that the animal has already been diagnosed with the disease clearly has a high probably of affecting the interpretation of ultrasonography findings. Of particular concern are study designs that ensure that the operator knows the entire clinical history (including previous test results) before conducting the ultrasonography. Ideally operators are unaware of the history. The direction of the bias caused by incorporation would be to increase the Se and Sp. Reports of Se and Sp that are based on post hoc analysis of hospital records from cases where no attempts have been made to conceal the clinical history are likely to be susceptible to incorporation bias. The following example illustrates an approach to study design that has a low risk of bias caused by incorporation bias. In a previous feedlot study focusing on ultrasonographic findings in naturally occurring BRD, the ultrasonographic examination was performed by the same operator who stored the pictures. The ultrasonograms were then randomized and read offline by a veterinarian who was blind to BRD status, as well as blind to the clinical appearance of the animal when the ultrasonography was performed.[22] The specific challenges concerning ultrasonography are that, when applied and interpreted calf-side or cow-side, the operator who is conducting the test cannot ignore the physical appearance of the animal, which in turn would have an effect on his/her interpretation of the examination. As a practical example, one can easily see that it is possible to interpret differently the same thoracic ultrasonographic picture/loop in a calf with depression, severe nasal discharge, and dyspnea, than in a calf without any apparent clinical sign of respiratory disease.

Classification bias

Classification bias occurs when the reference test is not a gold standard. If the reference test classifies some cases incorrectly, and Se and Sp are calculated based on the reference test, then incorrect estimates of true Se and Sp will occur. For example, if the index test is more sensitive than the reference test, then true positives based on the index will be classified as false-positives and result in decreased estimates of Sp. One solution for classification bias is to use latent class methods to estimate Se and Sp if the study design allows this.[23] This can be done using multiple imperfect tests including ultrasonography to assess their accuracy concerning the latent variable. This approach was used recently for assessing clinical scoring and thoracic ultrasonography accuracy in the diagnosis of BRD in dairy calves.[24] The specific challenge of the Bayesian latent class analysis is in the assessment of the robustness of the findings based on various previous assumptions (optimistic or pessimistic), especially when the number of animals is small.[25] Important modeling issues to be assessed include concern eventual conditional dependence between the tests, and constant accuracy of the tests in the subpopulations to be studied.[26]

Biases in Imaging Studies as a Result of the Approach to Conducting the Flow of Patients Through the Study

Partial verification and differential verification

It is obvious that all patients should be assessed by index (ultrasonography) and reference test(s); however, this is not always the case in some studies of diagnostic tests. In some studies, the decision to have the second test may be related to the results of the first. For example, a larger proportion that test positive on the first test are sent for a second opinion ultrasonogram. This bias is referred to as partial verification. When trying to assess the accuracy of echocardiography for the diagnosis of bovine endocarditis, it is apparent that cows that present undulating fever and heart murmur should be more systematically referred to cardiac ultrasonography examination than cows without heart murmur. The impact of this is usually that Se is increased and Sp is decreased.

Differential verification occurs when the reference test used is different between cases. For example, some cases may be considered positive based on clinical examination and radiographic (or necropsy) results, but because of costs (or side effects) not all animals would undergo radiography (or require euthanasia). In these situations, the animals would be considered cases based solely on clinical examination. This is referred to as differential verification bias. For example, in an earlier study describing thoracic diseases, the final diagnosis was based on physical examination in 21 cases and based on physical and necropsy examination in 33 cases.[27] These types of bias are often seen in studies that are post hoc analyses of hospital data, that is, 2-gate case-control studies. In a former 1-gate study on BRD in dairy calves, the investigators included up to 10 preweaned calves in the participating farms (among all the calves present at the day of the visit, starting from the oldest when more than 10 calves were present), which were systematically (no other selection filter) assessed by the 2 tests (thoracic ultrasonography and clinical scoring).[28] All the included calves had the same testing strategy used in case definition (although in this study ultrasonography was used as the reference standard and therefore does have some classification bias) and the cross-classification was performed at the end of the data collection.

Loss to follow-up bias or indeterminate results

Indeterminate results are those that are not clear. As can be intuitively expected, removing these patients can make the results look more conclusive. The reality is that some cases will not be 100% clear. Approaches to this problem include setting a cut-off for continuous outcomes. This should be determined before conducting the study and have a rationale. Other approaches are to conduct a sensitivity analysis and determine the differences in Se and Sp that would arise based on the treatment of the unclear cases as either positive or negative. For example, in a study focusing on application of ultrasonography for the diagnosis of BRD, not mentioning or eliminating cases where ultrasonography was inconclusive because of high body condition score (fatty animals), where poor ultrasonography quality was noted or did not include all cases where ultrasonography could not be performed safely (ie, wild or aggressive animals) could artificially inflate the test accuracy because of exclusion of cases where the index test may be inefficient.

Bias assessment or bias knowledge is therefore a critical issue when studying or designing ultrasonographic accuracy studies for medical and surgical interventions

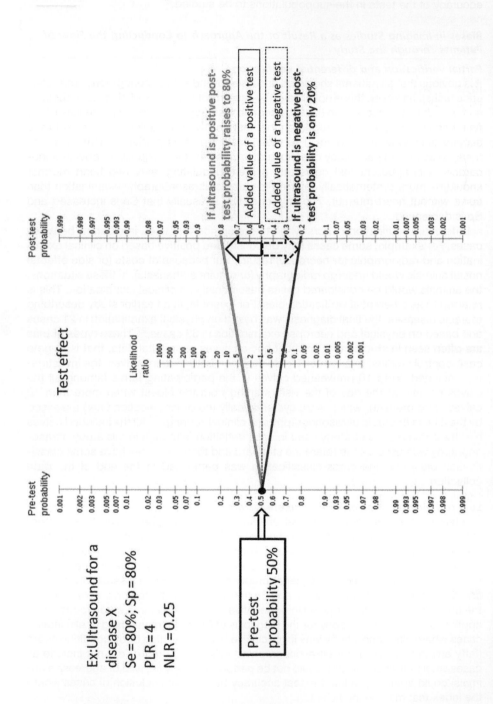

in cattle. This may also help the veterinarian to understand correctly the current knowledge and the weaknesses concerning this ancillary test for a specific diagnosis. The next step after the study has been completed and reported is to translate the results of the study in terms that can be easily understood and be applicable by the practitioner (ie, end user).

HOW TO PUT THE INCREMENTAL GAIN OF ULTRASONOGRAPHY OVER TRADITIONAL METHODS OF DIAGNOSIS TO PRACTICAL USE

As mentioned earlier, it is of crucial importance that evidence-based assessment of a diagnostic test encompasses the traditional Se/Sp assessment. However, even if it is considered as the last step in a diagnostic accuracy study, it is difficult to perform a randomized controlled trial on imaging tests in veterinary medicine. To the authors' knowledge, no randomized control trial has been published on an imaging diagnostic test in veterinary medicine to assess the "clinical value" of ultrasonography by comparing the change in case outcome when ultrasonography is or is not performed. This approach is also performed infrequently in human medical tests and shows the incremental gain when testing versus not testing (or vs current testing strategy).

Another appealing and clinically intuitive way to assess the diagnostic gain of a diagnostic test is to use the Fagan nomograms and Bayes theorem.[29] When obtaining Se and Sp of ultrasonography for a disease from a study at low risk of bias (or from future systematic reviews/meta-analysis of published studies), one can easily derive the LRs of a positive or negative result (see **Table 1**).

Based on the suspicion of disease before performing the test and the test results, the clinician can upgrade the new probability of disease (post-test probability) based on Bayes theorem[29]:

$$Odds_{Post-test} = Odds_{Pre-test} \times LR \tag{1}$$

with disease odds = $p/(1 - p)$, p = probability of the disease; so when replacing the odds by p:

$$p_{Post-test} = LR \times p_{Pre-test}/(1 - p_{Pre-test} + LR \times p_{Pre-test}) \tag{2}$$

As a practical example, we use the concept of a dairy cow with a 1-month history of undulating fever, tachycardia, and heart murmur. Before performing the test, one could easily guess, based on clinical experience, that the pre-test probability of having a bacterial endocarditis would be greater than 50%, and the echocardiographic examination would be positive. In a recent meta-analysis, we found that using echocardiography Se to detect bacterial endocarditis had wide confidence intervals (from 39.1%

◄―――

Fig. 2. Use of the Fagan nomogram and Bayes theorem to assess the practical accuracy of ultrasonography used as a diagnostic test. The practitioner needs to produce some values of sensitivity (Se), specificity (Sp), or negative or positive likelihood ratio (NLR, PLR). Based on the information before performing the test (clinical examination and empiric background with this type of case), the clinician has a rough pre-test suspicion of the disease (pre-test probability). The pre-test probability is then indicated in the Fagan nomogram (here 50%) as well as the PLR (if the test is positive) or NLR (if the test is negative). The line defined by the pre-test probability value and the corresponding LR is drawn and crosses the post-test probability line at the value of the post-test probability for this particular case (here 80% if the test is positive and 20% if the test is negative).

to 98.6%)[30]; the Sp was considered high but not calculated in that study (let us imagine that it was between 80% and 90% specific).

When considering a 50% pre-test probability, an Se/Sp value of 39.1/80, the positive likelihood ratio (PLR = 39.1/20 = 1.955) and negative likelihood ratio (NLR = 60.9/80 = 0.761) can be derived from **Table 1** by replacing Se and Sp by 0.391 and 0.80 which, when applying Equation 2 with the PLR (indicating that the ultrasonography finding results are positive) will lead to a post-test probability of disease of 66% (ie, 2 of 3 chances). If the ultrasonography results are negative, the post-test probability of endocarditis would only have decreased to 43% (so maybe still an indication to not rule out endocarditis). Using this approach allows us to see the practical incremental gain of the test (defined as the difference between post-test probability and pre-test probability; here 66–50, so a 16% increase after cardiac ultrasonography gives a positive result).

If our pre-test suspicion is increased to 60% in the case of a positive echocardiography, our suspicion would increase to 75% or decrease to only 53% in the case of a negative echocardiography (which may mean that we still need another test to rule in or rule out the disease). In the more optimistic scenario concerning accuracy of echocardiography (Se/Sp of 98.6/90), the test becomes much more informative (with PLR and NLR values of 9.86 and 0.016, respectively). Using a pre-test probability of 50%, a positive echocardiography would increase the post-test probability to 94%. In the case of a negative result, this probability would drop to only 2.3% (rejecting endocarditis would be true with a type 1 error $P<.05$).

The arithmetic behind these calculations may seem to be not very intuitive for the veterinary practitioner. To avoid these calculations, several graphic or online methods have been reported. Among these methods, the Fagan diagram can easily summarize the incremental gain of a test when the Se/Sp of the test is known (and therefore PLR and NLR) (**Fig. 2**).[31]

Even if not formally assessed in terms of precise numbers during day-to-day clinical practice, the practitioner is always intuitively using this type of approach because it is based on physical examination and anamnesis, and there is an analogy to previously seen cases and experience, which then leads to diagnostic testing and re-updating

---

Box 1
Several online calculators of pre-test and post-test probability based on test results (assessed on September 1, 2015)

- DocNomo app: a graphical tool to calculate LRs and post-test probability using sensibility and specificity for iOS devices https://itunes.apple.com/us/app/docnomo/id901279945?mt=8

- http://araw.mede.uic.edu/cgi-bin/testcalc.pl Diagnostic test calculator - Alan Schwartz (Web site). Allows computing post-test probability based on pre-test probability, test sensitivity, and specificity or LR with the graphical Fagan nomogram.

- http://www.kardiolab.ch/BayesCompact_e.html Web site that allows calculation of post-test probability based on test results and test accuracy. Web site difficult to go through and not very intuitive

- http://www.sample-size.net/post-probability-calculator-test-new/ Web site that allows the post-test probability to be calculated based on the pre-test probability and the likelihood ratio of the test

- https://www.easycalculation.com/statistics/post-test-probability.php Web site that allows the post-test probability to be calculated based on the pre-test probability and positive or negative likelihood ratio

the probability of disease according to the test result. The practical use of these calculations is to be able to quickly quantify the added value of the test by incorporating previously reported Se/Sp/PLR/NLR values from DTA studies with low risk of bias. We have added an excel spreadsheet to avoid these calculations (Appendix 1) as well as online calculators (**Box 1**).

In conclusion, there are several challenges to take into account when planning, performing, and reporting accuracy studies of diagnostic tests using ultrasonography for bovine medical and surgical disorders. We have information suggesting that ultrasonography may be efficient in the diagnosis of various ruminant diseases. The added value in terms of accuracy of implementation of ultrasonography in the routine diagnostic process still needs to be thoroughly studied and reported for many common ruminant diseases so that it may be more widely disseminated as an elegant way to improve diagnosis. Quantifying this improvement is a specific challenge that needs to be addressed, avoiding various types of biases that can occur in accuracy studies of diagnostic tests.

SUPPLEMENTARY DATA

Supplementary data related to this article can be found online at http://dx.doi.org/10.1016/j.cvfa.2015.09.009.

REFERENCES

1. Buczinski S. The information available on the use of ultrasound as an ancillary test continues to grow in peer-reviewed publications concerning experimental and clinical studies. Vet Clin North Am Food Anim Pract 2009;25:xi–xii.
2. Freedman LS. Evaluating and comparing imaging techniques: a review and classification of study designs. Br J Radiol 1987;60:1071–81.
3. Fei DY, Shung KK, Wilson TM. Ultrasonic backscatter from bovine tissues: variation with pathology. J Acoust Soc Am 1987;81:166–72.
4. Braun U, Pusterla N, Wild K. Ultrasonographic findings in 11 cows with a hepatic abscess. Vet Rec 1995;137:284–90.
5. Liberg P, Jonsson G. Ultrasonography and determination of proteins and enzymes in blood for the diagnosis of liver abscesses in intensively fed beef cattle. Acta Vet Scand 1993;34:21–8.
6. Rutjes AW, Reitsma JB, Vandenbroucke JP, et al. Case-control and two-gate designs in diagnostic accuracy studies. Clin Chem 2005;51:1335–41.
7. Lijmer JG, Mol BW, Heisterkamp S, et al. Empirical evidence of design-related bias in studies of diagnostic tests. J Am Med Assoc 1999;282:1061–6.
8. Bossuyt PM, Reitsma JB, Bruns DE, et al. Towards complete and accurate reporting of studies of diagnostic accuracy: the STARD initiative. Ann Intern Med 2003; 138:40–4.
9. O'Connor A, Evans RB. Critically appraising studies reporting assessing diagnostic tests. Vet Clin North Am Small Anim Pract 2007;37:487–97.
10. Buczinski S, Forté G, Bélanger AM. Short communication: ultrasonographic assessment of the thorax as a fast technique to assess pulmonary lesions in dairy calves with bovine respiratory disease. J Dairy Sci 2013;96:4523–8.
11. Bernier Gosselin V, Babkine M, Gains MJ, et al. Validation of an ultrasound imaging technique of the tympanic bullae for the diagnosis of otitis media in calves. J Vet Intern Med 2014;28:1594–601.
12. Resnick MI, Smith JA Jr, Scardino PT, et al. Transrectal prostate ultrasonography: variability of interpretation. J Urol 1997;158:856–60.

13. Geleijnse ML, Krenning BJ, van Dalen BM, et al. Factors affecting sensitivity and specificity of diagnostic testing: dobutamine stress echocardiography. J Am Soc Echocardiogr 2009;22:1199–208.
14. Whiting PF, Rutjes AW, Westwood ME, et al. QUADAS-2: a revised tool for the quality assessment of diagnostic accuracy studies. Ann Intern Med 2011;155: 529–36.
15. Higgins J, Altman D, Sterne J. Chapter 8: Assessing risk of bias in included studies. In: Higgins J, Green S, editors. Cochrane handbook for systematic reviews of interventions. Copenhagen, Danemark: Cochrane Collaboration; 2011. p. 1–50.
16. O'Connor A. Reporting guidelines for primary research: Saying what you did. Prev Vet Med 2010;97:144–9.
17. Santaguida PL, Riley CM, Matchar DB. Assessing risk of bias as a domain of quality in medical test studies. In: Chang SM, Matchar DB, Smetana GW, et al, editors. Methods guide for medical test reviews. Rockville (MD): Agency for Healthcare Research and Quality Publication; 2012. p. 67–76.
18. Kelly S, Berry E, Roderick P, et al. The identification of bias in studies of the diagnostic performance of imaging modalities. Br J Radiol 1997;70:1028–35.
19. Willis BH. Spectrum bias–why clinicians need to be cautious when applying diagnostic test studies. Fam Pract 2008;25:390–6.
20. Buczinski S, Tolouei M, Rezakhani A, et al. Echocardiographic measurement of cardiac valvular thickness in healthy cows, cows with bacterial endocarditis, and cows with cardiorespiratory diseases. J Vet Cardiol 2013;15:253–61.
21. Tharwat M, Oikawa S. Ultrasonographic evaluation of cattle and buffaloes with respiratory disorders. Trop Anim Health Prod 2011;43:803–10.
22. Abutarbush SM, Pollock CM, Wildman BK, et al. Evaluation of the diagnostic and prognostic utility of ultrasonography at first diagnosis of presumptive bovine respiratory disease. Can J Vet Res 2012;76:23–32.
23. Baker SG. A latent class method for diagnostic tests: the new, reference, gold standard problem. Stat Med 2014;33:4320.
24. Buczinski S, L Ollivett T, Dendukuri N. Bayesian estimation of the accuracy of the calf respiratory scoring chart and ultrasonography for the diagnosis of bovine respiratory disease in pre-weaned dairy calves. Prev Vet Med 2015;119:227–31.
25. Branscum AJ, Gardner IA, Johnson WO. Estimation of diagnostic-test sensitivity and specificity through Bayesian modeling. Prev Vet Med 2005;68:145–63.
26. van Smeden M, Naaktgeboren CA, Reitsma JB, et al. Latent class models in diagnostic studies when there is no reference standard–a systematic review. Am J Epidemiol 2014;179:423–31.
27. Flock M. Diagnostic ultrasonography in cattle with thoracic disease. Vet J 2004; 167:272–80.
28. Buczinski S, Forté G, Francoz D, et al. Comparison of thoracic auscultation, clinical score, and ultrasonography as indicators of bovine respiratory disease in preweaned dairy calves. J Vet Intern Med 2014;28:234–42.
29. Akobeng AK. Understanding diagnostic tests 2: likelihood ratios, pre- and post-test probabilities and their use in clinical practice. Acta Paediatr 2007;96:487–91.
30. Buczinski S, Tsuka T, Tharwat M. The diagnostic criteria used in bovine bacterial endocarditis: a meta-analysis of 460 published cases from 1973 to 2011. Vet J 2012;193:349–57.
31. Caraguel CG, Vanderstichel R. The two-step Fagan's nomogram: ad hoc interpretation of a diagnostic test result without calculation. Evid Based Med 2013;18: 125–8.

On-Farm Use of Ultrasonography for Bovine Respiratory Disease

Theresa L. Ollivett, DVM, PhD[a],*, Sébastien Buczinski, DrVét, DES, MSc[b]

KEYWORDS

- Calf pneumonia • Thoracic ultrasonography • Diagnostic tests • Consolidation
- Lung lesions • Ultrasonography scoring • BRD subtypes

KEY POINTS

- The portable rectal ultrasonography machines used by bovine veterinarians for reproductive examinations are a fast, accurate, and practical means of diagnosing the lung lesions associated with bovine respiratory disease (BRD) in young cattle.
- When combined with respiratory scoring, thoracic ultrasonography (TUS) allows the differentiation of the following subtypes of BRD: upper respiratory tract disease, clinical pneumonia, and subclinical pneumonia; all of which can be performance limiting.
- Poor prognostic indicators, including caudal lung lobe consolidation, lung abscessation, and lung necrosis, can be identified by TUS.
- TUS can be used at the herd level to identify specific populations at risk for developing BRD and to monitor the prevalence and severity of BRD over time, as well as any responses to management changes such as ventilation, vaccination, or changes in treatment protocols.
- A systematic TUS technique is imperative and must be based on anatomic and ultrasonographic landmarks.

INTRODUCTION

Clinical scoring systems have been developed over recent years to improve early and accurate detection of young cattle affected by bovine respiratory disease (BRD).[1,2] These systems are useful but fail to differentiate between upper and lower airway disease and do not identify calves with subclinical pneumonia. Radiography, computed tomography (CT), and ultrasonography (US) are noninvasive methods of diagnosing

---

The authors have nothing to disclose.
[a] Department of Medical Sciences, University of Wisconsin-Madison School of Veterinary Medicine, UW-SVM Room 2004, 2015 Linden Drive, Madison, WI 53706, USA; [b] Department of Clinical Sciences, Faculté de médecine vétérinaire, Université de Montréal, CP 5000, St-Hyacinthe, Québec J2S 7C6, Canada
* Corresponding author.
E-mail address: ollivett@wisc.edu

pneumonia antemortem. One retrospective study of 42 clinically ill adult dairy cows showed that the sensitivity (Se = 94%) of radiography was excellent, but specificity (Sp = 50%) was poor for identifying thoracic lesions compared with postmortem findings.[3] There was a high correlation (r = 0.94) between CT and postmortem levels of consolidation in young dairy calves after experimental infection with *Mannheimia haemolytica*.[4] However, radiography and CT are not practical for diagnosing pneumonia in large numbers of calves in a farm setting because of physical equipment constraints, expense, anesthetic requirements, and the potential for exposure to radiation. However, thoracic US (TUS) can be performed calf-side using portable, readily available machines without the fear of exposure to radiation.

This article reviews the existing relevant literature regarding TUS in young cattle, reviews the pertinent respiratory anatomy and systematic ultrasonographic examination with landmarks, and discusses practical on-farm applications for bovine practitioners.

ACCURACY OF THORACIC ULTRASONOGRAPHY IN YOUNG CATTLE

The pathophysiology of pneumonia is such that cellular infiltrates and cellular debris effectively displace air from the lung tissue,[5] resulting in nonaerated and/or consolidated lung lesions that are detectable by TUS. These lesions change the ultrasonographic character of the lung from that of a strong reflector with reverberation artifact to a homogeneous, hypoechoic structure similar to that of the liver[6] and allow the diagnosis of pneumonia regardless of the clinical state of the animal.[7,8]

Although diagnostic US has been available for more than 50 years, few studies were performed in dairy cattle during the first 20 years and none involved US of the lungs.[9] Since the early 1990s, more studies have focused on evaluating the accuracy of TUS for identifying the lung lesions associated with pneumonia. Three studies have purposefully calculated the diagnostic Se and Sp, whereas others have more generally correlated the association between TUS and postmortem examination.

The first study to assess TUS accuracy was performed using 18 Holstein-Friesian calves up to 5 months of age.[10] These calves had various stages of clinical bronchopneumonia, lung abscess, and/or pneumothorax, and were subjected to euthanasia because of the severity of the lung disease (n = 10) or polyarthritis (n = 8). The 12th intercostal space (ICS) to the third ICS were evaluated using a 7.5-MHz sector scanner and the location of each US lesion was documented by its location within the ICS relative to the surrounding bony landmarks (ie, hip, shoulder, and elbow). The lesions were then classified into 5 different categories based on the character and depth of the echogenic pattern: radiating artifacts, consolidations, fine-grained structure, medium-grained structure, and coarse-grained structure. A Se of 85% and Sp of 98% were reported after comparing results from TUS and gross postmortem examination. A 10-cm pulmonary abscess, a pneumothorax, and 1 case of interstitial pneumonia were not detected by TUS.[10]

More recently, we used bayesian analysis to estimate the sensitivity and specificity of TUS in 2 different commercial populations of preweaned Holstein calves.[11] BRD was highly prevalent in the Canadian population (n = 106) and of average prevalence in the second, American, population (n = 85). Landmarks used to complete the examination were as described previously.[10] However, instead of 5 categories of ultrasonographic lesions, calves were considered BRD positive when at least 1 cm of ultrasonographic consolidation was present. In addition, the TUS was performed using a portable, linear, 6.2-MHz rectal scanner instead of a higher frequency sector scanner. The estimated Se of TUS was 79.4% (bayesian credible intervals [BCI], 66.4–90.9) and the Sp was 93.9% (BCI, 88.0–97.6).

In 1998, Rabeling and colleagues[10] report a high accuracy of TUS. This finding comes despite failure to scan the cranial aspect of the right cranial lung, which is the most commonly affected lung lobe in dairy calves (Ollivett, unpublished data, 2012). The Se would have been much lower had cases of subclinical pneumonia been evaluated because lung lesions are often localized to the cranial aspect of the right cranial lobe.[12] Informative priors, or best guesses by a panel of experts, were used by Buczinski and colleagues[11] to model Se and Sp in the absence of a gold standard.

A third study reported Se and Sp of 94% and 100%, respectively, in 24 calves.[8] This study did assess the cranial aspect of the right cranial lung. However, this study evaluated the accuracy of TUS in detecting subclinical lung lesions, because only clinically normal calves were included. One calf had an atypical consolidated lesion located on the dorsomedial aspect of the right lung. This finding, in addition to the abscess undetected by Rabeling and colleagues,[10] highlights that lung lesions can only be detected ultrasonographically when they extend to the pleural surface.

Other studies have evaluated the general correlation between TUS findings and gross postmortem findings. One study assessed ultrasonographic lung lesions after an experimental bacterial infection with *Pasteurella multocida*.[13] There was excellent agreement between the postmortem examination and US distribution of lesions; however, only 1 postchallenge TUS scan was performed 48 hours after inoculation. More recently, Ollivett and colleagues[7] showed a high correlation ($r = 0.92$) between the amount of consolidated lung identified on TUS and gross postmortem examination.

Agreement between observers has also been evaluated. In a veal calf setting, 3 observers with varying levels of experience imaged 10 preweaned dairy calves (healthy, n = 4; treated for BRD, n = 6).[14] Skill levels ranged from experienced in TUS, experienced in extragenital US but not in TUS, and novice in any form of US. Depending on the experience level, the interobserver agreement was moderate to almost perfect (kappa = 0.6–1.0).

IMPLICATIONS OF ULTRASONOGRAPHIC LUNG LESIONS

Data are mixed for the short-term and long-term impacts of ultrasonographic lung lesions in young cattle. One study was unable to detect a measureable difference in average daily gain (ADG) in feedlot steers diagnosed with ultrasonographic lung lesions using a focused TUS in the third, fifth, and seventh right ICS and frozen images interpreted offline.[15] In a recent case-control feedlot study using a case definition with clinical signs, fever ($\geq 40°C$ [104°F]) and *M haemolytica* levels greater than 10^5 colony-forming units per milliliter of bronchial lavage fluid, TUS findings in BRD cases (maximal depth of consolidation, maximal area of consolidation and total consolidated area, number of sites with consolidation) were associated with the outcome (death) in the 15 days following enrollment.[16] However, the affected animals were not treated on the day of diagnosis or during the observation period. In dairy calves, lung lesions were associated with a lower body weight at 6 weeks of age,[17] reduced preweaning ADG of 45 g/d (0.10 lb/d),[18] and a potential for increased mortality.[19,20] The differences between the beef and the dairy studies likely reflect a difference in diagnostic Se between the TUS techniques used as well as differences in the life stage of the animals affected. The heavy forelimb muscles of postweaned beef calves or squeeze chute design preclude a complete examination of the cranial aspect of the cranial lung.

ULTRASONOGRAPHIC EQUIPMENT

In previous reports, ultrasound probe frequency and design included 3.5 MHz sector,[15] 3.5 to 13 MHz linear,[21,22] 7.5 MHz sector,[10] and 5 MHz convex.[23] Probe design is an important factor to consider when imaging the cranial thorax. Probes designed for transcutaneous uses are bulky. In contrast, transrectal probes permit better access to the axillary region and cranial thorax. They are also widely used by bovine veterinarians, making them most suitable for practical field-based TUS in young cattle. The operator can choose between using a machine with an attached screen, a wireless screen, or goggles, based on personal preferences.

CALF PREPARATION AND RESTRAINT

Operator positioning, restraint, and transducing agents are all necessary considerations when scanning. During the examination, it is up to the operator to decide whether to stand or squat down next to the calf (**Fig. 1**). Short individuals and those with low back pain typically prefer squatting, whereas those with knee pain or who are tall often choose to stand. When standing, it is easiest to scan each side of the calf by reaching over the dorsum to the opposite side. Feedlot calves can be examined in a squeeze chute with removable sections, which allows assessing the caudoventral part of the thorax.[16]

In most situations, restraint should be minimal, rarely requiring a halter, headlock, or chute, particularly in young dairy animals. Increasing the level of restraint often increases handling time, therefore reducing the practicality of the procedure. Most often, young dairy calves can be restrained by placing the hindquarters in the corner and a hand under the chin or in front of the chest. In headlocks, calves often lean backwards, reducing access to the first few ICS beneath the forelimb. Chutes can create dangerous obstructions and care should be taken in the positioning of the operator's arm when reaching inside to scan. Precautions should be taken as necessary when this becomes unavoidable in some older dairy and beef animals. On the farm, 70% isopropyl alcohol is the transducing agent of choice and the hair is not clipped or shaved from the chest. Ninety percent (or greater) isopropyl alcohol functions well but is excessively drying to the US probe as well as the skin of both the operator

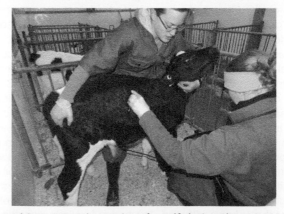

Fig. 1. Operator position. Manual restraint of a calf during thoracic US examination. The decision to squat next to the calf (as pictured) or stand is the preference of the ultrasonographer, but should be consistent.

and the calf, and should be avoided. Coupling gel and even vegetable oil work; however, both products create a substantial mess compared with alcohol. It is possible to screen greater than or equal to 30 calves with 1 gallon of alcohol after the operator has gained experience in using a typical large-bore squirt bottle or backpack sprayer (**Fig. 2**). Significantly less alcohol is required if a household spray bottle is used. Operators should not worry about exposing the probe to alcohol.

APPROACH

Technique is critical and veterinarians should be wary when presented with results from TUS studies in which the technique is not well described. In young cattle, the lung fields extend cranioventrally from the 10th to the first ICS on the right and the second ICS on the left, with most pneumonia lesions developing cranial to the 6th ICS. The US studies performed in the past examined the third to 11th or 12th ICS,[13,23] the 5th to 12th ICS,[24] or the right third, fifth, and seventh ICS.[15] Others only evaluated the seventh to 11th ICS.[22,25] Flöck[22] described bronchopneumonia as occurring predominantly in the cranioventral portions of the lung; however, the described technique only evaluated the lung lobes caudal to the seventh ICS, therefore excluding the left cranial lobe, the right middle lung lobe, and the right cranial lobe.

Within reason, the TUS technique can be modified based on the goals of the examination. When performing an US scan on an individual animal, the goal should be to evaluate the entire lung field on both the right and left sides. This goal requires scanning the right lung from the 10th ICS cranial to the first ICS and the left lung from the 10th ICS cranial to the second ICS (**Fig. 3**). Individual animals that are sick or doing poorly are more likely than average calves to harbor lesions, specifically lung abscesses, in the caudal lung lobe. In these cases, the caudal lung lobe should always be assessed.

When screening a group of calves for pneumonia, a different approach can be taken compared with that used for an individual sick animal. In this situation, TUS is used to screen specifically for bronchopneumonia. Bronchopneumonia reliably localizes to 3 specific lung lobes particularly during the early phase of disease. The cranial aspect of the right cranial lung lobe is most commonly affected, followed by the right middle lung lobe, and the caudal aspect of the left cranial lung lobe. The caudal aspect of the right cranial lung lobe, the cranial aspect of the left cranial lobes, and caudal lung lobe

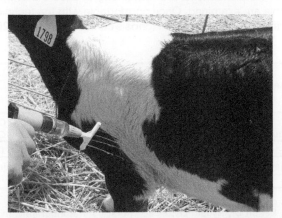

Fig. 2. Application of isopropyl alcohol using a commercially available drencher with a T-bar applicator. Drenching backpacks are useful when scanning large groups of calves.

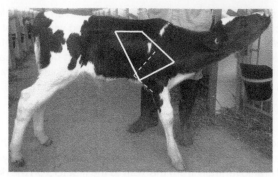

Fig. 3. Lung field outlined by solid white line in a preweaned Holstein dairy calf. The elbow is outlined by a dashed line. The elbow approximates the right middle or the caudal aspect of the left cranial lung lobes.

are rarely consolidated without consolidation of the previously mentioned lobes. It is important to scan both sides of the thorax because consolidation may occur unilaterally in up 1 in 3 dairy calves.[20] When a systematic clinical score, such as the Wisconsin Respiratory Score,[1] is also incorporated, calves can be categorized by BRD subtypes, including upper respiratory tract infections, clinical pneumonia, and subclinical pneumonia. In this context, upper respiratory infection is defined as a positive respiratory score and a normal TUS, clinical pneumonia is defined by a positive respiratory score and abnormal TUS, and subclinical pneumonia is defined by a normal respiratory score and an abnormal TUS. The distributions of BRD subtypes vary from farm to farm.

THORACIC ULTRASONOGRAPHY TECHNIQUE

The key to accurate TUS is being systematic. A systematic approach depends on an understanding of the external thoracic anatomy of the calf, the internal anatomy of the lung, and appropriate ultrasonographic landmarks (**Tables 1** and **2**). The external anatomy of the calf refers to the specific ICS where the probe is placed. The internal anatomy refers to the specific lung lobes that are being evaluated. The ventral image landmarks provide unique identifiers for each lung to ensure that the high-risk locations for pneumonia are examined. Once comfortable with the technique and scoring system, an accurate ultrasonographic diagnosis can be made within 20 to 30 seconds.

Table 1				
Landmarks for the right lung during ultrasonographic examination				
	Lung Lobe			
	Caudal	Middle	Caudal Aspect of Cranial Lobe	Cranial Aspect of Cranial Lobe
R-ICS	6–10	5	3–4	1–2
Ventral Landmarks	Diaphragm	CCJ and pleural deviation	Heart	Internal thoracic artery and vein

Abbreviations: CCJ, costochondral junction; R-ICS, right ICS.

From Ollivett TL, Kelton DF, Nydam DV, et al. Thoracic ultrasonography and bronchoalveolar lavage fluid analysis in Holstein calves affected with subclinical lung lesions. J Vet Intern Med. Accessed August 30, 2015. http://dx.doi.org/10.1111/jvim.13605. [Epub ahead of print.]

Table 2
Landmarks for the left lung during ultrasonographic examination

		Lung Lobe	
	Caudal	Caudal Aspect of Cranial Lobe	Cranial Aspect of Cranial Lobe
L-ICS	6–10	4–5	2–3
Ventral Landmarks	Diaphragm	CCJ and pleural deviation	Heart

Abbreviation: L-ICS, left ICS.
From Ollivett TL, Kelton DF, Nydam DV, et al. Thoracic ultrasonography and bronchoalveolar lavage fluid analysis in Holstein calves affected with subclinical lung lesions. J Vet Intern Med. Accessed August 30, 2015. http://dx.doi.org/10.1111/jvim.13605. [Epub ahead of print.]

In general, the recommended TUS examination extends from the caudal thorax to the cranial thorax by moving the probe along the grain of the hair in a dorsal to ventral fashion within each ICS (see **Fig. 1**). The probe should move parallel to the rib within the ICS. It is a common mistake to move the probe perpendicular to the ground. Instead, the probe should be moved slightly caudally, staying within 1 ICS to avoid imaging the rib. Very slight adjustments can move the ultrasound beam onto or off the rib surface and/or enhance visualization of a lung lesion. These small movements include moving the tip (or the end) of the probe side to side or rotating the footprint (the portion of the probe in contact with the body wall) so that it is facing more cranial or caudal within the ICS. If the rib obscures the image of the lung, stop moving, readjust the angle of the probe until the lung is present, and then continue ventrally within the ICS.

When scanning the right and left caudal lung lobes from the 10th to the sixth ICS, the diaphragm marks the ventral border of the lung. In this location, the liver can be seen deep to the diaphragm on the right (**Fig. 4**). The spleen is imaged deep to the

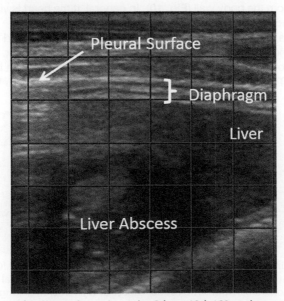

Fig. 4. Ultrasonographic image from the right 6th to 10th ICS at the ventral border of the right caudal lung lobe as denoted by the diaphragm and liver.

diaphragm on the left. In the general population of young cattle, bronchopneumonia is rarely present in the caudal lung lobes. However, focal pulmonary abscesses form in this location. Based on clinical experience, abscessation (ie, cavitary lesions with a discreet capsule) and the presence of consolidation that extends into this region typically carry a poor prognosis. Lung necrosis also carries a poor prognosis; however, necrosis is typically imaged more cranially in the usual sites for bronchopneumonia.

The right middle lung lobe is imaged from the right fifth ICS, whereas the caudal aspect of the left cranial lung lobe can be imaged between the left fourth to fifth ICS. In both locations, the ventral image landmark includes the pleural interface, which dives deep within the image as the costochondral junction appears ventrally (**Fig. 5**). The elbow roughly approximates the location of the fifth ICS. Bronchopneumonia commonly localizes to these lung lobes.

The caudal aspect of the right cranial lung lobe is imaged from the right fourth and third ICS. The heart is the ventral image landmark in both of these locations (**Fig. 6**). Expect to visualize only 1 to 2 footprints of lung in this location. If only the heart is imaged, the probe should be moved dorsally within the ICS. When affected by lobar pneumonia, a clear wedge-shaped lesion is easily appreciated.

The cranial aspect of the right cranial lung lobe is imaged from the right second and first ICS. These two locations image similarly, having an obvious step in the pleural interface as the lung moves around the internal thoracic artery and vein (**Fig. 7**). The pleural step and 2 vessels serve as the ventral image landmark on the right side. This position is the most common location for bronchopneumonia in dairy calves. However, it is the most difficult location to access for novice ultrasonographers. A couple suggestions will help ease the frustration associated with imaging this part of the lung. Holding the probe with the tips of 2 or 3 fingers of the left hand (**Fig. 8**), place it under the triceps muscle at the level of the middle third of the distance between the top of the scapula and the point of the elbow (**Fig. 9**), then slide it forward keeping the footprint flat against the thorax under the triceps without allowing it to slip and face away from the body wall (**Fig. 10**). In general, if the heart is visible, the probe should be advanced further cranially.

On the left side, the cranial aspect of the left cranial lung is imaged mainly from the third to the second ICS where the heart is the ventral image landmark. It is uncommon to image pneumonia here. Occasionally, a small amount of lung can be imaged from the left first ICS. This area is difficult to image and rarely adds useful information to the

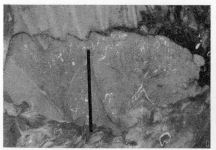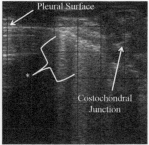

Fig. 5. Gross specimen and ultrasonographic image from the right fifth ICS at the ventral border of the right middle lung lobe (*black line*) as denoted by the pleural line diving deep under the costochondral junction. The caudal aspect of the left cranial lung images similarly from the left side. The lungs are grossly normally despite a few areas of pleural roughening (comet-tail artifacts) visible ultrasonographically. *Asterisk* denotes comet-tail artifact.

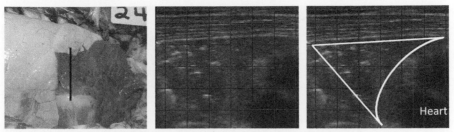

Fig. 6. Gross specimen and ultrasonographic image of the caudal aspect of the right cranial lung lobe (*black line*) as imaged from the right fourth ICS and affected by hypoechoic, lobar consolidation. The image would be nearly identical if scanned from the third ICS. The heart is the ventral image landmark in both locations.

examination, therefore operators are not compelled to scan. Of note, the cranial aspect of the right cranial lung can be imaged as it crosses the thorax in front of the heart from the left second ICS (**Fig. 11**). Occasionally, when just the tip is consolidated, it can be imaged only from this location. Access to the cranial aspects of the right and left cranial lung lobes is typically restricted to cattle less than 6 months of age.

ULTRASONOGRAPHY SCORING

Studies often measure the depth of the ultrasonographic consolidation over several locations on the thorax. It has been determined that the maximum depth of consolidation is well correlated with the number of locations with consolidation.[20] It makes

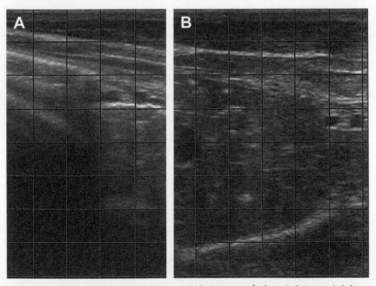

Fig. 7. Ultrasonographic images of the cranial aspect of the right cranial lung lobe as imaged from the first ICS on the right. Reverberation artifact and a hyperechoic pleural interface define the normal, aerated lung (*A*). A hypoechoic, lobar lesion indicates full-thickness consolidation of this lung lobe (*B*). The 2 blood vessels and step in the pleura marking the ventral landmarks are apparent on the right side of both images. The image would be similar if scanned from the second ICS but there would be more of a slope in the pleura around the vessels instead of a defined step down.

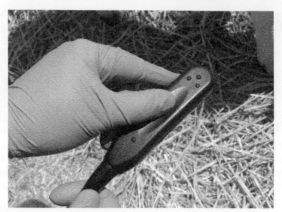

Fig. 8. Hand position when advancing the probe under the triceps muscle to examine the 2 portions of the cranial lung lobe.

anatomic sense that, as the depth of consolidation increases, the dorsal extent of the lesion increases, resulting in a similar increase in the number of sites with consolidated lung.

Counting centimeters of ultrasonographic lesions is not the fastest or the most practical method of grading TUS examinations for field veterinarians, especially when a grid option is not available on the unit, but can serve for research purposes to quantify more properly the amount of consolidated lung parenchyma. Categorical scoring systems are easier and more practical in the field. A 6-point scoring system (**Fig. 12**) is suggested and has served as a practical means to document and monitor lung lesions on commercial dairy farms for the author (TO).

In order to properly score, operators must be able to recognize the difference between aerated lung, aerated lung with diffuse pleural roughening (also called comet-tail artifacts), lobular lung lesions (also called lobular consolidations or lobular pneumonia), and lobar lung lesions (also called lobar consolidations or lobar pneumonia). Veterinary pathologists often use lobular pneumonia to describe a suppurative

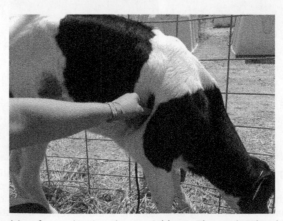

Fig. 9. Starting position for evaluating the cranial lung. The probe should be placed under the triceps muscle at the level of the middle third of the distance between the top of the scapula and the point of the elbow.

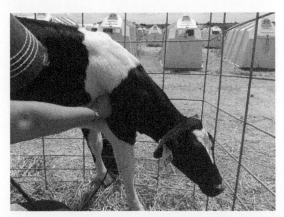

Fig. 10. Proper probe placement under the triceps muscle for examining the cranial aspect of the cranial lung.

bronchopneumonia caused by *P multocida* infection and lobar pneumonia to describe the more severe fibrinous pneumonia caused by *M haemolytica*.[26] In the context of the US scoring system outlined in **Fig. 12**, lobular and lobar lesions reflect the extent of which the lung lobe is consolidated on the US image. Lobular lesions are small

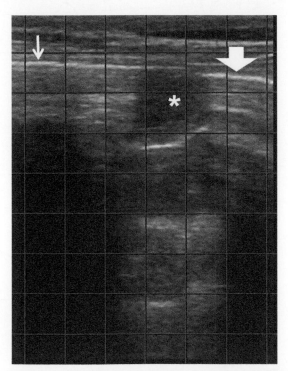

Fig. 11. Ultrasonographic image of both lungs taken from the left second ICS. The thick arrow indicates the right lung. The thin arrow indicates the left lung. The asterisk marks the thymus. Do not confuse the thymus with hypoechoic consolidation. Rarely, the thymus is visible ventrally in the first ICS on the right.

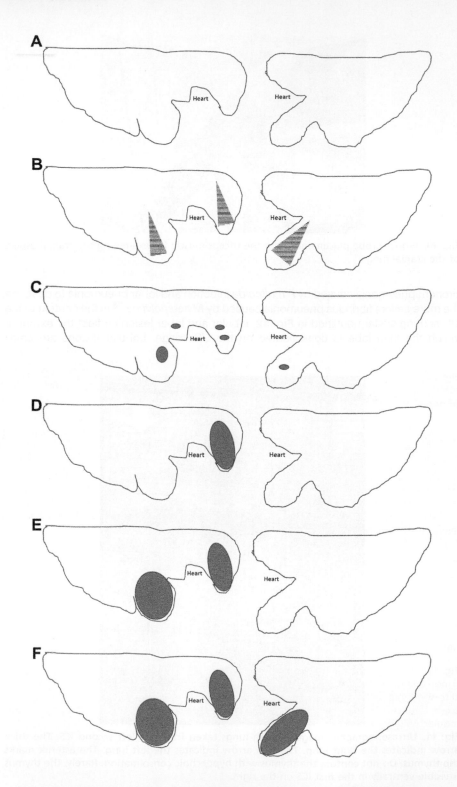

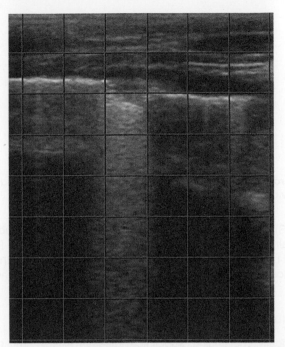

Fig. 13. Typical single lobular lesion imaged as small discreet area of consolidation within an otherwise aerated lung lobe. The hyperechoic pleural interface with reverberation artifact of normal lung is visible both dorsal and ventral to the lesion.

discreet areas of consolidation within an otherwise aerated lung lobe. The hyperechoic pleural interface with reverberation artifact of normal lung can be seen both dorsal and ventral to the lobular lesion when the probe is placed vertically within the rib space (**Fig. 13**). Lobar lesions indicate full-thickness consolidation of the lung lobe that extends proximally from the tip of the lobe. In the US image, the hypoechoic parenchyma of the entire distal lung lobe is visible, and aerated lung cannot be seen ventral to the lesion (see **Figs. 6** and **7**).

In general, US scores 0 to 1 are considered normal and US scores greater than or equal to 3 are consistent with bacterial bronchopneumonia.[8] Abnormalities such as pneumothorax, pleural fluid, abscesses, and necrosis are not inherently included in the scoring system. Instead, a comment is included within the record regarding the abnormality (eg, US score 4 plus 4-cm abscess in right caudal lung lobe at the level

---

Fig. 12. Ultrasonographic scoring system (0–5) used to categorize young cattle. (*A*) US score 0 indicates normal aerated lung with no consolidation and none to few comet-tail artifacts. Ultrasonographically, normal lung appears as a bright white, or hyperechoic, line. (*B*) US score 1 indicates diffuse comet-tail artifacts without consolidation. (*C*) US score 2 indicates lobular or patchy pneumonia. Small lobular lesions are most likely to be viral in nature and may not warrant treatment. (*D*) US score 3 indicates lobar pneumonia affecting only 1 lobe. (*E*) US score 4 indicates lobar pneumonia affecting 2 lobes. The cranial and caudal aspects of the cranial lobe are scored individually. (*F*) US score 5 indicates lobar pneumonia affecting 3 or more lobes.

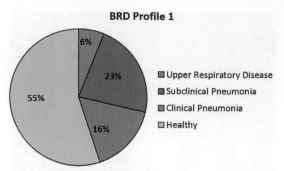

Fig. 14. Typical profile for BRD subtypes from a Wisconsin dairy milking 2700 cows with calves raised individually indoors.

of the eighth ICS). All US data are recorded calf-side using the publically available UW-Madison Calf Health Scoring iPad application. Data are stored for 1 year within the App and can be filled out as an Excel spreadsheet via e-mail at the user's discretion. If desired, scores can be manually entered into the cow files of the herd management software.

INDICATIONS AND IMPLEMENTATION

BRD is economically challenging, subclinical disease exists,[8] and producer-based diagnoses lack sensitivity.[11,27] Therefore, monitoring BRD in young cattle should be considered a priority for maintaining proper drug use, animal well-being, and profitability. However, bovine veterinarians are notoriously poor at doing so. Incorporating TUS at regular intervals not only provides an understanding of the epidemiology of BRD in client herds but more importantly helps to identify problems before they become catastrophic.

An astute German veterinarian commented once that it made the most sense to take TUS to her most progressive, early adaptor clients, which makes excellent sense. These producers typically seek their practitioner's input, find data useful, and look forward to the information from a new diagnostic tool. When the opportunity presents, the first step in monitoring BRD at the herd level with TUS is to acquire a baseline

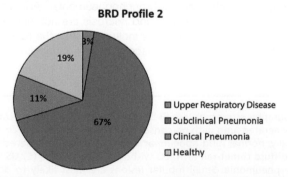

Fig. 15. Profile showing excessive subclinical pneumonia from a Wisconsin dairy milking 300 cows with calves raised in a new group housing facility with automatic feeders. Forty-eight percent of the subclinical cases scored greater than 3, indicating that 2 or more lung lobes were completely consolidated and necrotic lesions were visible in most.

Table 3
Example of how TUS can be used to measure the impact of a management change that took place during in late fall on a southern Wisconsin dairy. Clinical disease was based on respiratory score.[1] The presence of at least 1 moderately droopy ear defined otitis. Pneumonia was defined as score greater than or equal to 3 (see Fig. 12) using portable TUS. N = 160 Holstein calves in indoor group housing

	Summer 2014	Winter 2015	P Value
Clinical Respiratory Disease (%)	23	19	.25
Otitis (%)	21	11	.78
Pneumonia (%)	38	15	<.001

$P<.05$ indicates significant difference between variables across the row. Free software add-in for Microsoft Excel PopTools used for χ^2 test. http://www.poptools.org/.

of the calves at risk (on a small farm) or a random subset of calves at risk (8–12 calves could be a minimum number, although sometimes difficult to obtain in small herds, based on what has been recommended to assess herd metabolic health,[28] but larger numbers may be required when assessing an ongoing problem). Based on this information, along with clinical scoring, the distribution of the BRD subtypes (**Figs. 14** and **15**), age of onset, and duration of disease can be determined. The competency of animal care personnel can be assessed by calculating detection rates and the proportion of calves scoring greater than 3 (see **Fig. 12**) at first treatment. Detection rates are calculated by comparing the number of calves with pneumonia with daily treatment records and should be as high as 85%.[1] A high proportion of animals with lobar pneumonia affecting more than 1 lobe at first treatment suggests delayed detection and warrants additional training and protocol review with the employees. Excessive severe subclinical pneumonia (see **Fig. 15**) was present in a herd with poor detection, inadequate treatment regimen, inconsistent nutrition, and significant environmental challenges despite new facilities and acceptable stocking densities. TUS data help to measure the impact of management changes that are not reflected by changes in clinical signs or treatment records (**Table 3**, see **Figs. 14** and **15**).

SUMMARY

The portable rectal US machines already in use by bovine veterinarians for reproductive examinations are a fast, accurate, and practical means of diagnosing the lung lesions associated with BRD in young cattle. When combined with respiratory scoring, systematic TUS allows the differentiation of BRD into specific practical subtypes, including upper respiratory tract disease, clinical pneumonia, and subclinical pneumonia, all of which can be performance limiting. In individuals, TUS can be used to identify poor prognostic indicators such as caudal lung lobe consolidation, lung abscessation, and lung necrosis, and can aid culling and purchasing decisions. At the herd level, TUS can be used to identify specific populations at risk for developing the subtypes of BRD, to monitor the prevalence and severity of BRD over time, and to evaluate the impacts of management changes, such as changes in ventilation, vaccination, treatment protocols, or personnel. TUS can add to the services provided by bovine veterinarians, increasing their value and impact on animal health.

REFERENCES

1. McGuirk SM. Disease management of dairy calves and heifers. Vet Clin North Am Food Anim Pract 2008;24:139–53.

2. Love WJ, Lehenbauer TW, Kass PH, et al. Development of a novel clinical scoring system for on-farm diagnosis of bovine respiratory disease in pre-weaned dairy calves. PeerJ 2014;2:e238.
3. Masseau I, Fecteau G, Breton L, et al. Radiographic detection of thoracic lesions in adult cows: a retrospective study of 42 cases (1995-2002). Can Vet J 2008;49: 261–7.
4. Lubbers BV, Apley MD, Coetzee JF, et al. Use of computed tomography to evaluate pathologic changes in the lungs of calves with experimentally induced respiratory tract disease. Am J Vet Res 2007;68:1259–64.
5. Caswell JL, Williams K. Respiratory systems. In: Maxie MG, editor. Jubb, Kennedy, and Palmer's Pathology of domestic animals. 5th edition. Edinburgh (United Kingdom): Elsevier; 2007. p. 523–655.
6. Reef VB, Boy MG, Reid CF, et al. Comparison between diagnostic ultrasonography and radiography in the evaluation of horses and cattle with thoracic disease: 56 cases (1984-1985). J Am Vet Med Assoc 1991;198:2112–8.
7. Ollivett T, Hewson J, Schubotz R, et al. Ultrasonographic progression of lung consolidation after experimental infection with *Mannheimia haemolytica* in Holstein calves. J Vet Intern Med 2013;27:673.
8. Ollivett TL, Kelton DF, Nydam DV, et al. Thoracic ultrasonography and bronchoalveolar lavage fluid analysis in Holstein calves affected with subclinical lung lesions. J Vet Intern Med 2015. [Epub ahead of print].
9. Lamb CR, Stowater JL, Pipers FS. The first twenty-one years of veterinary diagnostic ultrasound. Vet Radiol Ultrasound 1988;29:37–45.
10. Rabeling B, Rehage J, Dopfer D, et al. Ultrasonographic findings in calves with respiratory disease. Vet Rec 1998;143:468–71.
11. Buczinski S, Ollivett TL, Dendukuri N. Bayesian estimation of the accuracy of the calf respiratory scoring chart and ultrasonography for the diagnosis of bovine respiratory disease in pre-weaned dairy calves. Prev Vet Med 2015;119:227–31.
12. Dagleish MP, Finlayson J, Bayne C, et al. Characterization and time course of pulmonary lesions in calves after intratracheal infection with *Pasteurella multocida* A:3. J Comp Pathol 2010;142:157–69.
13. Reinhold P, Rabeling B, Gunther H, et al. Comparative evaluation of ultrasonography and lung function testing with the clinical signs and pathology of calves inoculated experimentally with *Pasteurella multocida*. Vet Rec 2002;150:109–14.
14. Buczinski S, Forté G, Bélanger AM. Short communication: ultrasonographic assessment of the thorax as a fast technique to assess pulmonary lesions in dairy calves with bovine respiratory disease. J Dairy Sci 2013;96:4523–8.
15. Abutarbush SM, Pollock CM, Wildman BK, et al. Evaluation of the diagnostic and prognostic utility of ultrasonography at first diagnosis of presumptive bovine respiratory disease. Can Vet J 2012;76:23–32.
16. Rademacher RD, Buczinski S, Edmonds M, et al. Systematic thoracic ultrasonography in acute bovine respiratory disease of feedlot steers: impact of lung consolidation on diagnosis and prognosis in a case-control study. Bovine Pract 2014;48: 1–10.
17. Ollivett TL, Burton AJ, Bicalho RC, et al. Use of rapid thoracic ultrasonography for detection of subclinical and clinical pneumonia in dairy calves. In: Bob Smith, editor. St. Louis, MO: Proceeding of the American Association of Bovine Practitioners. Stillwater (OK): VM Publishing Company, LLC; 2011. p. 148.
18. Ollivett TL, Kelton DF, Duffield TF, et al. A randomized controlled clinical trial to evaluate the effect of an intranasal respiratory vaccine on calf health, ultrasonographic lung consolidation, and growth in Holstein dairy calves. In: Bob Smith,

editor. Albuquerque (NM): Proceedings of the American Association of Bovine Practitioners. Stillwater (OK): VM Publishing Company, LLC; 2014. p. 113–4.
19. Barringer S. Healthy calves: from birth to full ruminant. In: Bob Smith, editor. Albuquerque (NM): Proceedings of the American Association of Bovine Practitioners. Stillwater (OK): VM Publishing Company, LLC; 2014. p. 82–5.
20. Buczinski S, Forté G, Francoz D, et al. Comparison of thoracic auscultation, clinical score, and ultrasonography as indicators of bovine respiratory disease in preweaned dairy calves. J Vet Intern Med 2014;28:234–42.
21. Braun U, Sicher D, Pusterla N. Ultrasonography of the lungs, pleura, and mediastinum in healthy cows. Am J Vet Res 1996;57:432–8.
22. Flock M. Diagnostic ultrasonography in cattle with thoracic disease. Vet J 2004; 167:272–80.
23. Jung C, Bostedt H. Thoracic ultrasonography technique in newborn calves and description of normal and pathological findings. Vet Radiol Ultrasound 2004;45: 331–5.
24. Babkine M, Blond L. Ultrasonography of the bovine respiratory system and its practical application. Vet Clin North Am Food Anim Pract 2009;25:633–49.
25. Braun U, Pusterla N, Fluckiger M. Ultrasonographic findings in cattle with pleuropneumonia. Vet Rec 1997;141:12–7.
26. Panciera RJ, Confer AW. Pathogenesis and pathology of bovine pneumonia. Vet Clin North Am Food Anim Pract 2010;26:191–214.
27. Sivula N, Ames T, Marsh W, et al. Descriptive epidemiology of morbidity and mortality in Minnesota dairy heifer calves. Prev Vet Med 1996;27:155–71.
28. Oetzel GR. Monitoring and testing dairy herds for metabolic disease. Vet Clin North Am Food Anim Pract 2004;20:651–74.

Echocardiography for the Assessment of Congenital Heart Defects in Calves

Katharyn Jean Mitchell, BVSc, DVCS*,
Colin Claudio Schwarzwald, Prof Dr med vet, PhD

KEYWORDS

- Cardiac • Malformation • Bovine • Imaging • Ultrasonography

KEY POINTS

- Congenital heart disease in calves commonly presents as chronic respiratory disease, failure to thrive, or poor growth.
- The most common congenital heart disease in calves is a ventricular septal defect, either alone or in combination with more complex abnormalities.
- The prognosis for survival varies from guarded to poor and depends on the severity and hemodynamic relevance of the defects, but there is no specific prospective study in calves.

 Videos showing echocardiographic examples of congenital heart defects in calves accompany this article at http://www.vetfood.theclinics.com/

OVERVIEW

Congenital heart disease (CHD) in calves is uncommon, being observed in less than 0.2% of all bovine hearts inspected in 2 large necropsy studies.[1,2] A diagnosis of CHD is suspected following a history of ill thrift, poor growth, respiratory disease that fails to respond to appropriate therapy, and/or if a heart murmur is detected on physical examination.[3,4] Echocardiography is the most useful diagnostic test to confirm or rule out the presence of CHD. The detection of the common simple congenital abnormalities (eg, ventricular septal defects [VSDs]) is straightforward, but complex congenital abnormalities can prove more difficult to evaluate and interpretation of the images takes some experience and skill. Familiarity with the normal cardiac anatomy and a logical and standardized approach to the echocardiographic assessment are crucial to confirming a diagnosis of CHD. The authors recommend the

Disclosure: The authors have nothing to disclose.
Clinic for Equine Internal Medicine, Vetsuisse Faculty, University of Zurich, Winterthurerstrasse 260, Zurich 8057, Switzerland
* Corresponding author.
E-mail address: kmitchell@vetclinics.uzh.ch

Vet Clin Food Anim 32 (2016) 37–54
http://dx.doi.org/10.1016/j.cvfa.2015.09.002
vetfood.theclinics.com

systematic approach of sequential segmental analysis (SSA) when evaluating calves for CHD.[5]

EQUIPMENT AND SETTINGS

Echocardiography can be performed easily in calves in the field setting as well as the hospital. Despite the cranial location of the heart and the narrow intercostal spaces, echocardiography in calves is more rewarding than with adult cows.

Most calves can be evaluated using a medium-frequency probe (3.4–5 MHz) with a small footprint. A small, phased array probe is preferred, but microconvex, curvilinear, or linear probes can be used as well.

For two-dimensional echocardiography (2DE), the image should be optimized for a frame rate of at least 25 frames per second and typically 30 to 60 frames per second to fully appreciate cardiac motion. Higher frame rates can be achieved by reducing the sector width and imaging depth if necessary. An imaging depth of 10 to 15 cm is adequate for most young calves, whereas a depth of 15 to 20 cm may be necessary in older calves. Only 1 focal zone should be used, which is set to the far field. Tissue harmonics imaging results in a more favorable signal/noise ratio, increases depth of penetration, and improves endocardial border definition and visualization of cardiac structures, but echoes of fine structures such as valves and chordae appear thicker in harmonic imaging.

The 2DE-guided M mode uses a very high frame rate and therefore is capable of recording high-frequency motion (eg, a fluttering valve), which might be missed by the slower sampling rate of a 2DE study. Some echocardiography machines offer anatomic M mode, which can be used to derive M-mode tracings offline from 2DE cine-loop recordings and allows positioning of the M-mode cursor freely on the two-dimensional (2D) image, independent of the sector apex. However, this advantage can only be achieved at the expense of a lower temporal resolution, related to the low recording frame rate of 2DE recordings.[6]

In color Doppler imaging mode, a high frame rate (eg, achieved by narrowing the sector with and imaging depth), a slight reduction of tissue priority settings (favoring color priority), and selection of color maps with variance coding (eg, green coding of turbulent flow) facilitates recognition of intracardiac blood flow patterns. The velocity range is usually set near the maximum possible limits.

In spectral Doppler imaging mode (ie, pulsed-wave and continuous wave Doppler), the power can be reduced by 1 to 2 steps to increase clarity of the Doppler tracing, whereas specific filter settings allow the elimination of low-velocity noise. The velocity scale should be adjusted depending on the expected blood flow velocities to be recorded. More details on equipment and machine settings can be found elsewhere.[7]

A surface electrocardiogram (ECG) should be recorded simultaneously with all echocardiographic recordings for timing of cardiac events. If possible, cine loops containing at least 3 cardiac cycles should be recorded and stored. This method allows for offline measurements at several time points during the cardiac cycle and further evaluation of complex defects using slow motion playback. Still images are less optimal because subtle abnormalities may be difficult to detect.

PATIENT PREPARATION AND RESTRAINT

Young calves can be easily restrained in sternal or lateral recumbency, whereas older calves should be gently restrained standing. Most dairy breeds tolerate this procedure without sedation; however, light sedation may be necessary in older beef calves.

Clipping a small area (rectangle 8–10 cm) between the fourth and fifth intercostal spaces (immediately behind the elbow) on both sides of the chest improves the image quality. The skin can be gently cleaned with alcohol and ultrasonography coupling gel applied. If necessary, the thoracic limbs can be moved cranially to allow access to the relevant intercostal spaces.

IMAGING APPROACH/PROTOCOL

The technique for routine echocardiography in cattle is well described.[7–9] Familiarization with the normal anatomy and standard imaging planes for echocardiography is essential when attempting to diagnose CHD. In general, the imaging planes for calf echocardiography are similar to those required for equine and small animal echocardiography (**Fig. 1**).[7]

Right Parasternal Views

In a normal calf, most echocardiographic views are taken from the right parasternal imaging window. Long-axis 4-chamber, right ventricular outflow tract (RVOT) and left ventricular outflow tract (LVOT) imaging planes provide the basis for capture of the main cardiovascular structures (atria, ventricles, great vessels, atrioventricular [AV] and arterial valves) and subjective assessment of cardiovascular function. Short-axis 2D and M-mode images of the ventricles obtained at the level of the papillary muscle and chordae tendineae, mitral valve, left atrium (LA), and aorta (Ao)/ pulmonary artery (PA) provide additional morphologic and functional information. From there, color flow mapping and spectral Doppler analysis can help identify the presence of intracardiac shunting, valvular regurgitation, or any inflow or outflow tract obstruction.

Left Parasternal Views

The left parasternal imaging window can be useful for detecting left heart disease.[8] Long-axis views of the atria, ventricles, Ao, and in particular the main PA can be obtained. In the authors' experience, in some cases because of the positioning of the heart or concurrent lung disorder, the left parasternal window may provide better access to some or all of the cardiac structures.

Apical 4-Chamber/5-Chamber Views

Depending on the calf's size, an apical 4-chamber or 5-chamber view, similar to that used in human and small animal echocardiography, can provide superior alignment for color and spectral Doppler studies. These views are obtained by sliding the transducer near the apex close to the sternum and scanning dorsally and cranially to view all chambers. The 4-chamber view includes the LA, left ventricle (LV), right atrium (RA), and right ventricle (RV), whereas the 5-chamber view also includes the Ao.[7]

SEQUENTIAL SEGMENTAL ANALYSIS

The anatomy and spatial orientation of the cardiac chambers and great vessels can be markedly abnormal in many cases of complex congenital malformation. This abnormality makes interpretation of echocardiographic recordings difficult and often necessitates the use of unconventional imaging planes to display all the relevant cardiac structures.

Therefore, for echocardiographic assessment and diagnosis of CHD, the recommended approach in both human and veterinary echocardiography is SSA. All

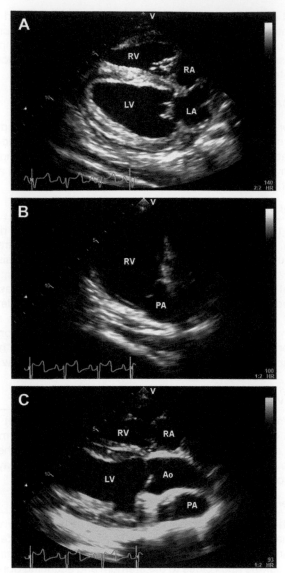

Fig. 1. 2D B-mode recordings in (*A*) right parasternal long-axis 4-chamber view, (*B*) right ventricular outflow tract (RVOT) view, (*C*) left ventricular outflow tract (LVOT) view, (*D*) right parasterna short-axis view at the level of the papillary muscles, and (*E*) left parasternal long-axis view. The base of the heart is to the right, the apex to the left of the screen in the long-axis images. An ECG is superimposed for timing. The red marker on the ECG tracing indicates the timing of the frame within the cardiac cycle. Ao, aorta; LA, left atrium; LV, left ventricle; PA, pulmonary artery; RA, right atrium; RV, right ventricle.

hearts, no matter whether normal or abnormal, are made up of 3 segments: atria, ventricles, and the great vessels (Ao and PAs). Using SSA, the orientation and relationship between cardiac segments are investigated in a stepwise fashion. The cardiac segments are identified based on their anatomic features and not their just spatial orientation.[5,10]

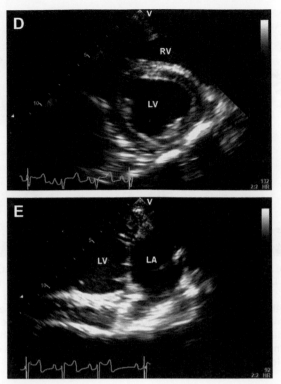

Fig. 1. (continued).

Step 1: Atrial Arrangement

Determining the presence and arrangement of the atria is the first step in SSA. The atria are best identified based on the morphology of their appendages. The morphologic RA is characterized by a broad-based, triangular appendage with the terminal crest and extensive pectinate muscles. The morphologic LA has a narrow-based, tubular appendage with no obvious terminal crest and less obvious pectinate muscles.

The arrangement of the atria can be described as usual (situs solitus), mirror imaged (situs inversus, reported in 5 cases in the literature[11]), right isomerism (morphologically bilateral right atria), or left isomerism (morphologically bilateral left atria). Partitioning of the atrial chambers can occur (cor triatriatum dexter or sinister) but is extremely rare with no cases reported in the literature. The authors have recognized one 2-month-old brown Swiss calf with cor triatriatum sinister (**Fig. 2**).

Step 2: Ventricular Arrangement

Assessment of the ventricular arrangement is the second step of SSA. The morphologic RV possesses coarse apical and septomarginal trabeculations, the leaflet of the atrioventricular (AV) valve attaches directly to the septum, and there is an obvious moderator band. The morphologic LV has fine apical trabeculations and a smooth upper part of the septum without attachments to the AV valve. Absence of a ventricular septum can result in a solitary, morphologically indeterminate ventricle.[11,12] The ventricles can be hypoplastic but complete (with developed inlet, trabecular, and outlet portions) or they can be hypoplastic and incomplete (rudimentary, often lacking the

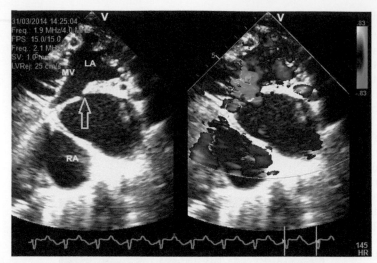

Fig. 2. 2D B-mode (*left*) and simultaneous color Doppler recording (*right*) of the left parasternal long-axis, LA view. This calf was diagnosed with cor triatriatum sinister. The LA is divided into 2 compartments with a narrow communication (*arrow*) from the upper compartment (with pulmonary veins draining into it) to the lower one (communicating with the LV and mitral valve (MV) and the RA via a large atrial septal defect [ASD]). Color flow mapping indicates turbulent flow (color coded in *green*) through the communication between compartments. Additional turbulent flow is seen in the lower LA compartment as a result of right-to-left shunting of blood across a large ASD.

inlet portion). There are several reports of calves with abnormal ventricular shape and arrangement in the literature.[11,13,14]

In cases with severe congenital malformations, it may be difficult to differentiate the LV and RV. Hypoplastic ventricles are often more easily detected. Failure to identify a rudimentary chamber is most indicative of a solitary, indeterminate ventricle.

Step 3: Atrioventricular Connections

The third step of evaluation is to describe the AV connections, by establishing how the atrial segments are connected with the ventricular mass. There are 3 main groups of AV connections.

Biatrial, biventricular connections may be considered concordant (atria connected to the appropriate ventricle), discordant (atria connected to the inappropriate ventricle), or ambiguous (eg, with atrial isomerism).

Biatrial, univentricular connections are present if the atria only connect to 1 ventricle, either as a double inlet AV connection (both atria connect with the same dominant ventricle), an absent right AV connection (only the LA is connected with the ventricular mass), or an absent left AV connection (only the RA is connected with the ventricular mass). These last 2 scenarios occur when 1 atrium ends blindly in a muscular floor at an AV junction (AV valve atresia). Usually, the connected ventricle is dominant and the nonconnected ventricle is hypoplastic and rudimentary, or a solitary ventricle exists.

Uniatrial, biventricular connections occur when a solitary AV connection straddles and overrides the ventricular septum, connecting the atrial mass to both ventricles.

A double inlet LV, an absent left AV connection, and 2 atria with a single ventricle have been reported in calves.[11,13,14]

Step 4: Morphology of the Atrioventricular Valves

The fourth step is to determine the morphology of the AV valves, independent of the AV junctional connections. There may be 2 AV valves, or just 1 common valve. The valves can be straddling and overriding, dysplastic (malformed), or partially or completely imperforate (atretic). The leaflets of the AV valves can have an abnormal length or shape, or they can be thickened, fenestrated, or fused. The papillary muscles and chordae tendineae might be altered with respect to shape, size, length, position, or orientation.

When investigating AV valve morphology, standard 2D images are most useful. The use of M mode can provide additional information to assess valve motion. Doppler studies can assist to identify regurgitation (turbulent systolic blood flow in the atria) or stenosis (high-velocity transvalvular diastolic blood flow, V_{max} >2 m/s). This combined information can help assess the type and severity of the malformation. A variety of AV valve abnormalities, usually in combination with other complex congenital defects, have been described in calves; however, tricuspid valve atresia has not been reported.[11]

Step 5: Ventriculoarterial Connections

This fifth step is extremely important in diagnosing complex malformations in calves because abnormal ventriculoarterial connections are frequently described in the literature.[12,13] When 2 great arteries are present (either normally developed or hypoplastic), the junction is termed concordant (arteries connected to the appropriate ventricles), discordant (arteries connected to the inappropriate ventricles; eg, transposition of the great vessels), or double outlet (both arteries arising from either the left, the right, or an indeterminate ventricle; eg, double-outlet RV [DORV]). These variations are shown in **Fig. 3**. An echocardiographic example of a calf with a DORV is shown in **Fig. 4** and Video 1.

The Ao and PA can be differentiated by identifying the coronary arteries, which always arise from the Ao, and the origin of the branching vessels (brachiocephalic trunk originating from the Ao, left and right PAs arising from the main PA).

If there is atresia of either the Ao or the main PA, this is termed single outlet, as is the presence of a single common or solitary arterial trunk. A common arterial trunk is characterized by a single arterial vessel arising from the base of the heart that gives rise to the systemic, pulmonary, and coronary circulation. In a solitary arterial trunk, the Ao and coronary arteries are identified but the PAs are absent and the pulmonary circulation is provided by systemic-pulmonary collaterals arising from the descending Ao.[12]

Visualization of the great vessels and their branches using echocardiography is crucial for the correct antemortem classification of the malformation, but this can be extremely challenging. If an atretic vessel is strandlike, it may be impossible to detect using echocardiography. A careful postmortem dissection is required to confirm the diagnosis in these cases.

Step 6: Morphology of the Arterial Valves

The morphology of the arterial valves is assessed in the sixth step. Overriding valves are assigned to the ventricle supporting more than 50% of their circumference. The valves can be normal (tricuspid) or they may contain an abnormal number of cusps (eg, bicuspid, quadricuspid). They can be dysplastic, hypoplastic, or atretic. The cusps may be thickened, fenestrated, or fused.

Similarly to the AV valves, the morphology and function of the arterial valves can be assessed using 2D and M-mode echocardiography and the presence of regurgitation and/or stenosis can be evaluated using Doppler studies.

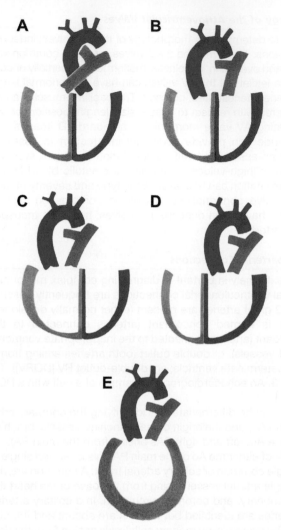

Fig. 3. (A) Concordant (normal) and (B) discordant (transposition) ventriculoarterial connections. The Ao is colored in red, the PA in blue. Double outlet can be from the (C) morphologically RV (*blue*), (D) morphologically LV (*red*), or (E) indeterminate ventricle (*purple*).

Step 7: Associated Malformations

In addition, the septal structures, outflow tracts, great arteries (including the arterial duct and the aortic arch), the coronary arteries, and the system and pulmonary venous connections should be assessed for malformation. Most of the described complex CHDs in calves have 1 or more of these abnormalities.[3,11]

SPECIFIC CONGENITAL MALFORMATIONS
Abnormal Communications (Shunts)

Atrial, atrioventricular, and ventricular septal defects

A thorough interrogation of all septal structures (atrial, AV, and ventricular) should be performed. The most common congenital defects reported in calves are ventricular

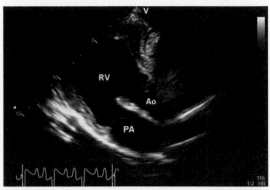

Fig. 4. 2D B-mode recording, right parasternal long-axis, RVOT view. This calf has a DORV; with both the Ao and PA visualized next to each other and connected with the RV.

septal defects (VSD), either alone or in combination with other complex malformations.[1,3,11] Abnormalities of the atrial and AV septa are also well documented, although much less common than VSDs.[11,15]

Interatrial communications are most commonly detected in combination with complex malformations but they also infrequently occur as isolated defects. They are divided into defects of the oval fossa (secundum-type atrial septal defects [ASDs]), cranial and caudal sinus venosus defects, and coronary sinus defects. Differentiation (with echocardiography) between a secundum-type ASD and a patent foramen ovale (PFO) can be difficult, especially with smaller defects. In the case of a PFO, the septal structures are fully developed but, because of high RA pressures (ie, pulmonary vascular disease), the flap of tissue covering the foramen ovale remains unfused and right-to-left shunting of blood can occur. Care should be taken not to overinterpret the echocardiography findings, because the oval fossa within the interatrial septum can appear anechoic in normal animals and Doppler studies can be confusing because of streaming of normal flow patterns (ie, caudal vena cava flow) overlying the interatrial septum. Saline contrast (bubble) studies can provide additional information and confirm right-to-left shunting of bubble-containing blood into the LA (**Box 1**). Even with this method, streaming of normal blood from the caudal vena cava may produce negative contrast in the RA, falsely suggesting left-to-right shunting of blood.[5,16] The common locations for interatrial communications are shown in **Fig. 5**.

Atrioventricular septal defects can be grouped into those that affect the interatrial component of the AV septum (ostium primum defects) and those that have a common AV canal with a common AV junction (endocardial cushion defects). The latter are usually large and easily detected with 2D echocardiography. AV septal defects have been infrequently detected in calves.[11]

Communications between the ventricles or VSDs can occur as isolated abnormalities or as part of a complex malformation. In general, VSDs are characterized according to the location and size. The defects can be located in the area of the membranous septum, adjacent to the right/noncoronary cusps of the aortic valve and the septal leaflet of the tricuspid valve (the most common type, termed perimembranous or paramembranous), immediately below the aortic and pulmonic valves (the less common type, termed subpulmonic, supracristal, subarterial, or doubly committed), or within the muscular part of the interventricular septum (rare type, termed muscular). The common anatomic locations for VSDs are identified in **Fig. 5**. Detection of VSDs using

Box 1
Saline contrast (bubble) study protocol

Materials

- Intravenous (IV) catheter placed in the right jugular vein
- IV extension set
- Three-way stopcock
- Use 20-mL of normal saline in a 20-mL syringe, connected to the 3-way stopcock
- Empty 20-mL or 30-mL syringe, connected to the 3-way stopcock

Procedure

- Use either the left or right parasternal long-axis view to image the region of interest (eg, interatrial or IVS with adjacent chambers). Agitate the saline for 30 seconds immediately before injection by moving it rapidly back and forth between the 2 syringes that are attached to the 3-way stopcock. Obtain a cine-loop recording immediately before, during, and for 10 to 15 seconds after injection of the agitated saline into the intravenous catheter. The agitated saline containing small air bubbles provides positive echo contrast and, if no cardiac shunts are present, the bubbles will only be present in the right heart (**Fig. 10**). If bubbles appear in the left heart shortly after injection, there must be some form of rightto-left shunting of blood, most commonly a VSD, ASD, or both (**Fig. 11**). If transpulmonary shunting through arteriovenous connections is present, a small number of bubbles might appear in the LA and LV only after a few heart beats (but not immediately after injection).

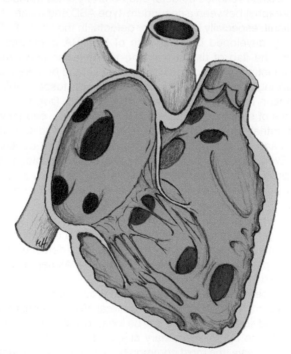

Fig. 5. The common locations of ASDs and VSDs. The largest blue area is the oval fossa, where true ASDs occur. The other, smaller blue areas are locations of other possible interatrial communications. The yellow area is the location of perimembranous VSDs. The orange area shows the location of subpulmonic VSDs. The green areas are possible locations for muscular VSDs in the inlet, apical, and outlet portions of the septum.

echocardiography is straightforward, although nonconventional views may be required in addition to the standard imaging planes. Color flow mapping may help detect small VSDs that are not clearly observed on the 2D images and care must be taken to screen the entire IVS from apex to base in long-axis and short-axis imaging planes for the presence of small muscular VSDs. Spectral Doppler recordings can assess peak shunt flow velocity, allowing estimation of the pressure gradient across the defect (**Box 2**).[5] Examples of perimembranous and subpulmonic VSDs are shown in **Figs. 6–8** and Videos 2–5. An example of an ASD is shown in **Fig. 9**.

Patent ductus arteriosus

In calves, the ductus arteriosus can remain patent following birth, as an isolated abnormality or in association with other malformations. In most normal calves, the ductus arteriosus should be functionally closed within the first few days of life.[11] It can be challenging to identify the arterial duct and ductal flow with 2D and color Doppler echocardiography, but assessment should include interrogation of several views of the main PA from both the right and left imaging windows. Spectral Doppler imaging may indicate disturbance of diastolic flow in the main PA in cases with significant left-to-right shunting of blood.

Aortopulmonary window

This term describes a communication between the great arteries in the setting of separate pulmonic and aortic valves. Differentiation should be made between an aortopulmonary window and a common arterial trunk, with a common trunk connected to the base of the ventricle via a single valve and a VSD present.[12] This defect has been reported once in calves.[11]

Box 2
Prognostic evaluation of VSDs

Estimation of the size of the VSD from 2D and color Doppler images:

- VSD to aortic root diameter ratio less than or equal to 0.3: small, restrictive VSD

- VSD to aortic root diameter ratio greater than or equal to 0.6: large, unrestrictive VSD

Estimation of the pressure gradient between RV and LV based on spectral Doppler velocity measurements across the VSD:

- Velocity greater than 4.5 m/s indicates a normal LV-to-RV pressure gradient of greater than 80 mm Hg

- Velocity less than 3.0 m/s indicates a decreased LV-to-RV pressure gradient of less than 36 mm Hg (caused by RV hypertension and/or LV hypotension)

Assess for evidence of pulmonary hypertension:

- Enlarged PA compared with Ao (PA/Ao ratio >1.0)

- High-velocity pulmonic insufficiency (>2.5 m/s if present)

- High-velocity tricuspid regurgitation (>3.2 m/s if present)

Assess for evidence of left-sided volume overload

- LA and LV enlargement

Note that these key points are based on current practice in equine cardiology and should provide a rough point of reference when applied to calves; published data to support prognostic factors associated with VSDs in calves are lacking.

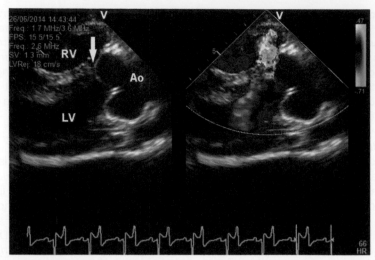

Fig. 6. 2D B-mode (*left*) and simultaneous color Doppler recording (*right*) of the right parasternal long-axis, modified LVOT view. A restrictive perimembranous VSD (*arrow*) is present. Color flow mapping indicates turbulent shunt flow (color coded in *green*) through the defect during diastole.

Outflow Tract Obstructions

Even in the absence of abnormal ventriculoarterial connections, attention should be paid to the outflow tracts of each ventricle. Stenosis of the outflow tract can be located in the subvalvular, valvular, or supravalvular regions. Subvalvular stenosis can result from shelves of fibrous tissue, muscular (septal) hypertrophy, or anomalous

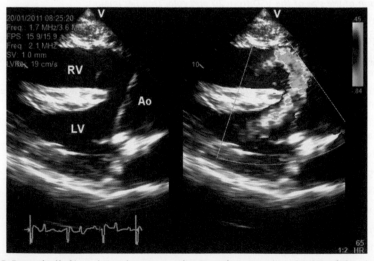

Fig. 7. 2D B-mode (*left*) and simultaneous color Doppler recording (*right*) of the right parasternal long-axis, modified LVOT view. A large perimembranous VSD is present concurrently with an enlarged overriding Ao. Color flow mapping indicates end-diastolic flow across the defect. This calf was diagnosed with a tetralogy of Fallot.

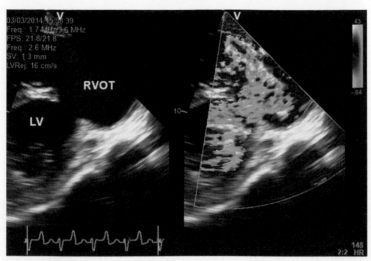

Fig. 8. 2D B-mode (*left*) and simultaneous color Doppler recording (*right*) of the right parasternal short-axis view at the level of the mitral valve. A large subpulmonic VSD is present, connecting the LV with the RVOT. Color flow mapping indicates turbulent shunt flow (color coded in *green*) through the defect during systole.

muscular bundles (hypertrophied septomarginal trabeculations). Valvular stenosis can result from hypoplasia or dysplasia of the valves with fusion, tethering, or thickening of the leaflets. Supravalvular stenosis can occur because of constriction of the sinotubular junction or diffuse hypoplasia of the great artery. Dynamic outflow obstruction may contribute to subvalvular stenosis as a result of muscular hypertrophy, accessory AV valve tissue prolapsing into the outflow tract, or anterior motion of the septal mitral leaflet during systole. Standard 2D and M-mode echocardiographic assessment allow evaluation of the ventricular outflow tracts, valve morphology, and motion. Spectral Doppler recordings can quantify the resulting hemodynamic consequences and allow estimation of the degree of stenosis (aortic and pulmonic outflow tract velocities >2 m/s [pressure gradients >16 mm Hg] can indicate stenosis).[5,7] To the authors' knowledge, isolated pulmonic or aortic stenosis has not been reported in

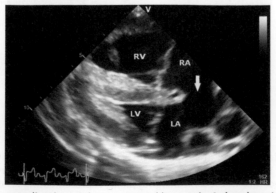

Fig. 9. 2D B-mode recording in a right parasternal long-axis, 4-chamber view focused on the atria. A large ASD is present (*arrow*), connecting the RA and the LA atrium.

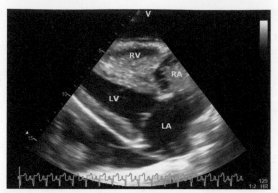

Fig. 10. 2D B-mode recording in a right parasternal long-axis, 4-chamber view. The image was captured while a saline contrast (bubble) study was being performed. The contrast is visible as hyperechoic content in the RA and the RV but not in the LA and LV. There is no evidence of an intracardiac shunt.

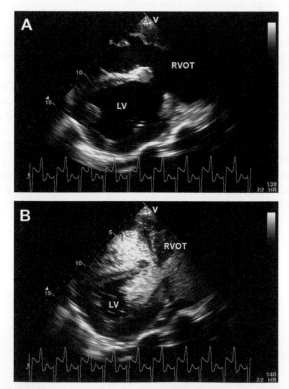

Fig. 11. 2D B-mode recording in a right parasternal short-axis view, below the level of the mitral valve. (*A*) A large subpulmonic VSD in its typical location, connecting the LV with the RVOT. (*B*) Image recorded in the same imaging plane, captured during a saline contrast (bubble) study. There is intense saline contrast present in the RV and the RVOT, extending through the defect into the LV, indicating diastolic right-to-left shunting across this large defect.

calves but may be detected in combination with other complex CHD abnormalities (eg, pulmonic stenosis with a tetralogy of Fallot).[11]

Tetralogy/Pentalogy of Fallot

A combination of pulmonic stenosis, right ventricular hypertrophy, and a VSD with an overriding Ao forms the complex known as tetralogy of Fallot. This form of CHD is well documented in calves, with more than 42 cases in the literature.[11,17,18] A severe form of this abnormality can be associated with pulmonic atresia.[19] If combined with an ASD, these abnormalities become a pentalogy of Fallot.

Coronary Abnormalities

Coronary artery anomalies can occur with variations in the site of origin, aberrant course, abnormal number, and fistulous communications between branches of the coronary arteries and a cardiac chamber or vessel. A large number of coronary artery variations have been described in calves. In contrast with humans, calves more often have an anomalous origin of the right coronary artery (originating from the pulmonary trunk).[11] Coronary artery–ventricular fistulas also dominated among other coronary artery abnormalities.[11] Echocardiographic detection of coronary abnormalities can be extremely difficult and even a postmortem diagnosis can be challenging in many cases.

Anomalies of Systemic and Pulmonary Venous Connections

These defects are considered rare in calves.[11] Examples include total or partial anomalous pulmonary venous return, persistent left cranial vena cava, or aberrant caudal venous return via the azygous vein. Echocardiographic assessment is difficult in most cases. Careful dissection in situ during a postmortem examination is required for a correct diagnosis.

Abnormalities of the Aorta and Aortic Arch

These defects are considered extremely rare in calves.[11] The most common is aortic tubular hypoplasia (described by some investigators as aortic coarctation or obstruction of the aortic arch usually at the level of the ductus arteriosus). An in vivo diagnosis via transthoracic echocardiography is often not possible.

Abnormal Heart Location

Ectopia cordis, mainly cervical, in which the heart is not appropriately contained within the thorax, is a frequently described condition in calves with more than 165 cases reported in the literature.[11] The clinical diagnosis is generally obvious in these cases. Occasionally, additional cardiac malformations are reported in these ectopic hearts.

HEMODYNAMIC CONSEQUENCES OF CONGENITAL HEART DISEASE

Following the echocardiographic description and diagnosis of the morphologic abnormalities, the hemodynamic consequences of the malformations need to be investigated in order to assess their clinical relevance and prognosis. With careful consideration, the blood flow patterns through the heart, including intracardiac shunting, and the pressure conditions in the cardiac chambers can be predicted based on the sequential segmental analysis and theoretic hemodynamic scenarios.

Real-time, 2D echocardiographic evaluation of the cardiac chamber dimensions, wall thickness, septal motion, and ventricular function are all important parts of the overall assessment of cardiac function and hemodynamic consequences. Saline contrast (bubble) studies (for more information see **Box 1**), color flow mapping, and spectral Doppler assessment allow further identification of blood flow streaming patterns and can be used to quantify intracardiac shunts, or evaluate inflow or outflow tract stenosis or valvular regurgitations.

Assessment of the Hemodynamic Relevance of Ventricular Septal Defects

At present, published data to support prognostic factors associated with VSDs in calves are lacking. However, information is available for horses and small animals and may be useful as a rough point of reference when assessing the hemodynamic relevance of a VSD in calves. Both the size of the defect and estimation of the pressure gradient across the defect have been used to determine whether the VSD should be considered restrictive or nonrestrictive.

Based on the equine literature, VSDs smaller than one-third of the aortic root diameter and with a left-to-right shunt velocity of greater than 4.5 m/s indicate restrictive physiology and are associated with normal performance and favorable prognosis.[20,21] In practice, calves with restrictive VSDs do not show clinical signs associated with CHD and are therefore often not recognized as such, unless a heart murmur is heard as an incidental finding. In contrast, defects with a VSD to aortic root diameter ratio of 0.6 or greater and with a left-to-right shunt velocity of less than 3.0 m/s, evidence of marked pulmonary overcirculation, and left-sided cardiac enlargement are hemodynamically relevant and associated with clinical signs of heart disease and a guarded to poor prognosis (see **Box 2**). Pulmonary hypertension may develop secondary to chronic pulmonary overcirculation as a result of the left-to-right shunting across the VSD. In advanced cases, increasing RV pressures can lead to reversal of the shunt flow, now being right-to-left across the VSD. This condition, termed Eisenmenger complex, is infrequently reported in calves with severe, hemodynamically relevant VSDs (see **Box 2**).[3]

PROGNOSIS AND OUTCOMES OF CONGENITAL HEART DISEASE

Clinically, patients with CHD present with one of 4 common groups of history or physical findings.

1. Failure to thrive/poor weight gain/chronic respiratory disease
2. Signs of cyanosis
3. Signs of congestive heart failure (right, left, or biventricular)
4. Heart murmur heard incidentally on physical examination

The patient's clinical presentation can also provide evidence for the hemodynamic consequences of the malformations that may be present. Typically, animals with severe, complex abnormalities are younger and often show signs of intracardiac shunting with cyanosis and respiratory distress, weakness, or failure to nurse. There are some lesions (eg, hemodynamically relevant VSDs) that take some time before clinical signs of disease are detected, because the heart's compensatory mechanisms play a delaying role in the onset of clinical signs. Cattle show a remarkable tolerance for severe congenital malformations, with some cases only detected in older calves, heifers, or adult cows. Note that cyanosis is only present in CHD leading to right-to-left shunting (ie, tetralogy of Fallot, transposition of the great arteries, truncus arteriosus, tricuspid atresia, and total anomalous pulmonary venous connection), but not in the most commonly seen VSDs with left-to-right shunting. Clinically, cyanosis may be difficult to detect in milk-fed calves with a low-iron diet. These animals are frequently anemic with resultantly low concentrations of desaturated hemoglobin, making the visual observation of cyanosis harder.

In most cases of CHD affecting calves, the advanced diagnostic work-up of complex congenital cardiac disease is largely of academic interest, because there is limited practicality to treatment or management of heart disease in cattle. An accurate diagnosis and assessment of the severity of disease may be important in individual cases with isolated defects (ie, restrictive VSDs), which can be associated with a favorable prognosis. However, severe and complex malformations are often associated with a hopeless prognosis for long-term productivity and survival.[3,22] If detailed information is required about the prognosis in a calf with CHD, referral to a veterinary cardiologist for a specialist evaluation is recommended. Note also that the hemodynamic consequences of less severe defects may take months to years to develop, and follow-up evaluations may be necessary to determine the presence and rate of disease progression.

SUPPLEMENTARY DATA

Supplementary data related to this article can be found online at http://dx.doi.org/10.1016/j.cvfa.2015.09.002.

REFERENCES

1. van Nie CJ. Congenital malformations of the heart in cattle and swine. A survey of a collection. Acta Morphol Neerl Scand 1966;6:387–93.
2. Hagio M, Murakami T, Tateyama S, et al. Congenital heart in disease in cattle. Bull Fac Agric Miyazaki Univ 1985;32:233–49.
3. Buczinski S, Fecteau G, DiFruscia R. Ventricular septal defects in cattle: a retrospective study of 25 cases. Can Vet J 2006;47:246–52.
4. Sandusky GE, Smith CW. Congenital cardiac anomalies in calves. Vet Rec 1981;108:163–5.
5. Schwarzwald CC. Sequential segmental analysis - a systematic approach to the diagnosis of congenital cardiac defects. Equine Vet Educ 2008;20:305–9.
6. Grenacher PA, Schwarzwald CC. Assessment of left ventricular size and function in horses using anatomical M-mode echocardiography. J Vet Cardiol 2010;12:111–21.
7. Boon J. Veterinary echocardiography. 2nd edition. Chichester, West Sussex: Wiley-Blackwell; 2011.
8. Buczinski S. Cardiovascular ultrasonography in cattle. Vet Clin North Am Food Anim Pract 2009;25:611–32.
9. Amory H, Jakovljevic S, Lekeux P. Quantitative M-mode and two-dimensional echocardiography in calves. Vet Rec 1991;128:25–31.
10. Carvalho JS, Ho SY, Shinebourne EA. Sequential segmental analysis in complex fetal cardiac abnormalities: a logical approach to diagnosis. Ultrasound Obstet Gynecol 2005;26:105–11.
11. Michaelsson M, Ho SY. Congenital heart malformations in mammals. London: Imperial College Press; 2000.
12. Ho SY, Rigby ML, Anderson RH. Echocardiography in congenital heart disease made simple. London: Imperial College Press; 2005.
13. Gopal T, Leipold HW, Dennis SM. Congenital cardiac defects in calves. Am J Vet Res 1986;47:1120–1.
14. Lemberger KY, Mohr KR, Andrews JJ. Atypical hypoplastic left ventricular syndrome in a calf. J Vet Diagn Invest 2004;16:423–6.

15. Murakami T, Hagio N, Hamana K, et al. Morphology of atrial septal defects in cattle. J Jpn Vet Med Ass 1991;44:696–9.
16. Steininger K, Berli AS, Jud R, et al. Echocardiography in Saanen-goats: normal findings, reference intervals in awake goats, and the effect of general anesthesia. Schweiz Arch Tierheilkd 2011;153:553–64.
17. Mohamed T, Sato H, Kurosawa T, et al. Tetralogy of Fallot in a calf: clinical, ultrasonographic, laboratory and postmortem findings. J Vet Med Sci 2004;66:73–6.
18. Suzuki K, Uchida E, Schober KE, et al. Cardiac troponin I in calves with congenital heart disease. J Vet Intern Med 2012;26:1056–60.
19. Nakade T, Uchida Y, Otomo K. Three cases of bovine extreme tetralogy of Fallot. J Vet Med Sci 1993;55:161–7.
20. Reef VB. Evaluation of ventricular septal defects in horses using two-dimensional and Doppler echocardiography. Equine Vet J 1995;27:86–95.
21. Reef VB, Bonagura J, Buhl R, et al. Recommendations for management of equine athletes with cardiovascular abnormalities. J Vet Intern Med 2014;28:749–61.
22. Buczinski S, Rezakhani A, Boerboom D. Heart disease in cattle: diagnosis, therapeutic approaches and prognosis. Vet J 2010;184:258–63.

Ascites in Cattle
Ultrasonographic Findings and Diagnosis

Ueli Braun, Prof Dr Med Vet, Dr Med Vet H C

KEYWORDS

- Cattle • Ultrasonography • Noninflammatory ascites • Inflammatory ascites
- Peritonitis • Uroperitoneum • Hemoperitoneum • Biliary ascites

KEY POINTS

- Ascites is excessive accumulation of fluid in the peritoneal cavity; based on clinical examination alone, this condition can be difficult to diagnose because signs of abdominal fluid accumulation may be subtle and detected only after careful examination.
- The identification of the cause of ascites can be demanding and undoubtedly is facilitated by an in-depth knowledge of physiology and internal medicine.
- Abdominocentesis and examination of the aspirated fluid are mandatory steps in the examination of an animal with ascites.
- Ultrasonography allows the assessment of the extent and nature of the fluid accumulation and also identifies other pathologic changes, including dilation of the cranial vena cava, severe liver lesions, bladder rupture, or fibrinous deposits on abdominal organs, that might point to the cause of the ascites.

INTRODUCTION

Ascites is excessive accumulation of fluid in the peritoneal cavity. Based on clinical examination alone, this condition can be difficult to diagnose because signs of abdominal fluid accumulation may be subtle and detected only after careful examination. Furthermore, the identification of the cause of ascites can be demanding and undoubtedly is facilitated by an in-depth knowledge of physiology and internal medicine. Abdominocentesis and examination of the aspirated fluid are mandatory steps in the examination of an animal with ascites. Ultrasonography allows the assessment of the extent and nature of the fluid accumulation and also identifies other pathologic changes, including dilation of the cranial vena cava, severe liver lesions, bladder rupture, or fibrinous deposits on abdominal organs, that might point to the cause of the ascites. Ultrasonography includes evaluation of the fluid as well as the various

The author has nothing to disclose.
Department of Farm Animals, University of Zurich, Winterthurerstrasse 260, CH-8057 Zurich, Switzerland
E-mail address: ubraun@vetclinics.uzh.ch

Vet Clin Food Anim 32 (2016) 55–83
http://dx.doi.org/10.1016/j.cvfa.2015.09.004   vetfood.theclinics.com

organ systems; therefore, special knowledge of the ultrasonographic features of these organs is an invaluable asset.

DIAGNOSTIC PROCEDURE IN SUSPECTED CASES OF ASCITES

The diagnostic procedure for ascites includes clinical examination, urinalysis, hematological and biochemical analysis of the blood, abdominal ultrasonography, and abdominocentesis. This article focuses on the ultrasonographic examination of the abdomen.

Clinical Examination

Clinical examination does not reveal ascites unless the abdominal fluid accumulation is pronounced, at which time pear-shaped enlargement of the abdomen, a strikingly flaccid abdominal wall, and sloshing of fluid on abdominal succussion are evident. The differential diagnosis includes conditions accompanied by fluid accumulation in the gastrointestinal tract or in the pregnant uterus. Whether the fluid is intraruminal, in the intestines, uterus, or the peritoneal cavity is determined during transrectal examination. Ascites accompanied by a tense abdomen, an arched back, and positive foreign body tests is suggestive of peritonitis with intraperitoneal exudate.

Blood Examination

This examination comprises hematological and biochemical analyses, including the measurement of the packed cell volume and white blood cell count and the concentration of serum total solids, fibrinogen, electrolytes, urea, creatinine and bilirubin and the activities of liver enzymes. The serum albumin concentration should always be determined in cattle with noninflammatory ascites.

Ultrasonographic Examination

Ultrasonography is a very sensitive, rapid, and accurate technique for the detection of peritoneal fluid.[1] Even very small amounts of fluid are readily visualized; the localization, extent, and nature of the peritoneal fluid can be assessed. In addition, it is often possible to identify the cause of the ascites.

Abdominocentesis

Abdominocentesis and examination of the aspirated fluid are required for the characterization of the ascites fluid, to differentiate noninflammatory and inflammatory ascites, and to distinguish between uroperitoneum, hemoperitoneum, chylous ascites, and bile peritonitis.

TECHNIQUES OF ABDOMINAL ULTRASONOGRAPHY AND ABDOMINOCENTESIS
Ultrasonography Technique in Suspected Cases of Ascites

Ultrasonographic examination is carried out on both sides of the abdomen and transrectally in the standing nonsedated animal.[2] The hair is clipped on both sides and the skin cleaned with alcohol before applying conductive gel. Linear or convex transducers with a frequency of 3.5 to 5.0 MHz are ideal, but abnormalities close to the abdominal wall can also be assessed with a 7.5-MHz transducer. The abdomen is examined on both sides from caudal to cranial. The transducer is placed at the paralumbar fossa and then moved ventrally to the midline. The intercostal spaces 12 to 7 are also examined with the transducer held parallel to the ribs. The urinary bladder and uterus are examined transrectally with the transducer directed ventrally, and the caudal part of the left kidney is examined with the transducer directed dorsally.

The abdominal organs normally occupy the entire abdominal cavity and are separated from each other and the peritoneum by capillary spaces, which contain very small amounts of serous fluid to lubricate the surface of tissues. The capillary spaces are not normally visible sonographically but can be imaged when they enlarge as a result of fluid accumulation or other disease processes. Likewise, the omentum and mesentery are difficult to visualize sonographically in healthy ruminants but are easily seen when outlined by fluid. The high fat content of these structures increases sound reflection. The organ contours usually are smooth, and echoic deposits with or without fluid inclusions are considered abnormal. The fluid between organs is assessed for amount and echogenicity; the latter can range from anechoic to echoic and may appear homogeneous or heterogeneous. With inflammatory ascites, echoic sediment may be seen at the lowest point accompanied by a hypoechoic or even anechoic supernatant. Gaseous inclusions generated by gas-producing bacteria may be seen as echoic stippling. Strands of fibrin can often be seen running in a spiderweblike fashion between organs or between an organ and the parietal peritoneum. Normal ultrasonographic findings have been published for the reticulum,[3] rumen,[4] omasum,[5] abomasum,[6] small intestines,[7] colon,[8] liver,[9] spleen,[10] and urinary tract.[11,12]

Technique for Abdominocentesis in Suspected Cases of Ascites

Abdominocentesis is ideally conducted under ultrasound guidance at a site where ultrasonographic changes are seen.[2] The site is clipped and the skin cleaned with alcohol and disinfected. After administering local anesthesia, a 20-gauge × 3.5-in spinal needle with stylet (0.90 × 90.0 mm, Terumo Spinal needle, Terumo Medical Corporation, USA) is inserted into the peritoneal cavity. Depending on the viscosity of the fluid, a larger-bore needle (18 gauge × 3.5 in, 1.20 × 90 mm) may be used. When the fluid appears heterogeneous, the collected sample should include parts of the echoic sediment to increase the likelihood of obtaining inflammatory or tumor cells and bacteria. The amount, color, transparency, odor, and consistency of the collected fluid are assessed; the presence of cellular or other material is noted (**Box 1**). A refractometer is used to measure specific gravity and total solids, and the California mastitis test is used to estimate the cell count. Cytologic and bacteriologic examinations are undertaken when the California mastitis test is positive. The urea and creatinine concentrations are measured when uroperitoneum is suspected.

When assessing aspirated peritoneal fluid,[13–16] it should be remembered that the classic differentiation of abdominal transudate and exudate does not always apply in sick cattle. A typical exudate is defined as cloudy, watery to viscous, foul-smelling fluid that may clot quickly after collection. An exudate often contains flecks of fibrin and pus.

Box 1
Goals of abdominocentesis

1. Assessment of amount, color, odor, and consistency of a sample (eg, serous, bloody, purulent, urinelike, bilelike)

2. Determination of specific gravity and concentration of total protein (total solids) using a refractometer

3. California mastitis test for semiquantitative determination of cellular content of fluid

4. Cytologic, bacteriologic, and possibly biochemical evaluation of fluid

5. Comparison of urea and creatinine concentrations of peritoneal fluid and serum

The specific gravity is greater than 1.015 and the protein content greater than 30 g/L. Smears made from exudates contain numerous leukocytes, but the number of cells may be reduced because of cytolysis. The proportion of eosinophils and neutrophils is used as a criterion for the diagnosis of peritonitis[14]; fewer than 10% eosinophils and greater than 40% neutrophils is highly suggestive of peritonitis. Sterile pus without bacteria may occur after antibiotic treatment of the animal, and the presence of bacteria in the absence of leukocytes may indicate contamination from accidental intestinal puncture. To improve the diagnostic usefulness of peritoneal fluid analysis, other variables, including albumin, glucose, fibrinogen, L-lactate, D-dimers, and the activities of lactate dehydrogenase and creatine kinase, were measured in serum and peritoneal fluid of 95 cows; the peritoneal-to-serum ratios of these variables were calculated.[17] The glucose concentrations of blood and peritoneal fluid are usually similar, but bacteria in the peritoneal cavity metabolize glucose and cause a decrease in the peritoneal glucose concentration. The glucose concentration is, therefore, considered a very sensitive and specific criterion for the diagnosis of septic peritonitis in cattle.[18] L-lactate is a metabolite of anaerobic glycolysis, and ischemic processes in gastrointestinal organs result in an increase in its concentration in peritoneal fluid and secondarily in blood.[18] D-dimer is a fibrin degradation product and plays an important role in the diagnosis of coagulation and thrombotic diseases. Healthy cattle have a D-dimer serum concentration of less than 0.60 mg/L.[17] Peritonitis in cattle is associated with massive synthesis of fibrin immediately accompanied by fibrinolysis, which generates D-dimer. D-dimer is considered the best criterion for the diagnosis of peritonitis.[17] Analogous to other species, a sensitivity of 96% and specificity of 98% was calculated for the D-dimer concentration in peritoneal fluid for the diagnosis of peritonitis in cattle.[18]

TYPES OF FREE PERITONEAL FLUID

There are many different types of peritoneal fluid (**Table 1**), including inflammatory, noninflammatory, chylous, urinelike, hemorrhagic, and bilious fluids. Small fluid accumulations may only be seen at the lowest point of the abdomen, but large accumulations involve the entire peritoneal cavity; the space between organs increases because of the fluid surrounding them. Because of the superb acoustic properties of fluid, the ultrasonographic visibility of organs suspended in fluid is better than the normal in situ appearance.

NONINFLAMMATORY ASCITES

Noninflammatory ascites is the abnormal accumulation of serous fluid in the peritoneal cavity.[2] An increase in intravascular hydrostatic pressure and/or a decrease in intravascular colloid osmotic (oncotic) pressure are the principal causes of

Table 1
Types and characteristics of intra-abdominal peritoneal fluid accumulation

Type of Intra-Abdominal Fluid	Characteristics
Inflammatory ascites	Exudate
Noninflammatory ascites	Transudate or modified transudate
Chylous ascites	Milky fluid
Uroperitoneum	Urinelike fluid
Hemoperitoneum	Bloody fluid
Biliary ascites	Bilious fluid

noninflammatory ascites. It is most commonly caused by vascular congestion but can also be the result of hypoalbuminemia (decrease in oncotic pressure), retention of sodium accompanied by water retention in secondary aldosteronism, or peritoneal cancer, such as mesothelioma.[19–22] Often the cause of noninflammatory ascites is multifactorial.

Clinical Signs of Noninflammatory Ascites

A tentative diagnosis can be made in severe cases when symmetric ventral abdominal enlargement causing a pear-shaped abdomen, a flaccid abdominal wall, and sloshing of fluid on abdominal succussion are evident (**Fig. 1**). When the condition is missed or allowed to continue, the contour of the animal may progress to barrel shaped (**Fig. 2**). Abdominal enlargement caused by ascites is generally more pronounced in calves and other young cattle than in mature cattle. However, even in cases with

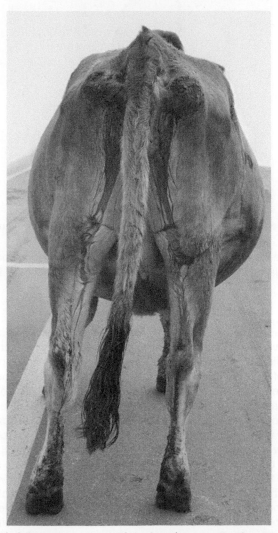

Fig. 1. Pear-shaped abdomen in a cow with ascites due to uroperitoneum.

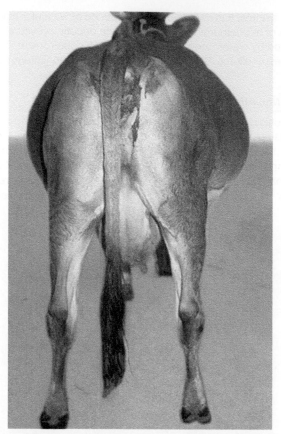

Fig. 2. Barrel-shaped abdomen in a cow with ascites due to uroperitoneum.

considerable intra-abdominal fluid accumulation, the pear-shaped abdominal appearance may be missed. Ultrasonography is the method of choice for diagnosis of ascites.

Ultrasonographic Findings of Noninflammatory Ascites

The typical ultrasonographic finding of noninflammatory ascites is accumulation of anechoic fluid of varying extent in the peritoneal cavity. It may be limited to the ventral abdomen or the fluid level may extend dorsally or involve the entire peritoneal cavity. Large amounts of fluid surround the organs so that they are suspended in it. On the right side, intestines enclosed by the greater omentum are seen from the flank and intercostal spaces (**Fig. 3**). The surrounding fluid renders the greater omentum echoic; both walls of the omental bursa, each consisting of 2 serous layers, can often be seen (**Fig. 4**). The liver is displaced dorsally by the fluid and seen in the costal part of the abdomen. However, with mild or moderate ascites, only the ventral part of the liver including the gall bladder is surrounded by fluid (**Fig. 5**). With severe ascites, the liver is displaced from the abdominal wall creating an anechoic seam between the parietal peritoneum and the liver. Hepatic ligaments are often seen as fine echoic strands between the liver and the abdominal wall. On the left side, the rumen is displaced from the abdominal floor by anechoic fluid (**Fig. 6**). Likewise, the reticulum is displaced dorsally by fluid (**Fig. 7**). Owing to the acoustic properties of peritoneal fluid, the

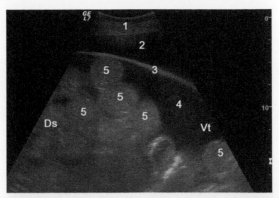

Fig. 3. Ultrasonogram of ascites in a cow with compression of the caudal vena cava by a liver abscess, imaged from the right flank. Loops of small intestine are displaced dorsally by anechoic ascites fluid. 1, lateral abdominal wall; 2, extraomental ascites fluid; 3, greater omentum; 4, intraomental ascites fluid; 5, small intestine. Ds, dorsal; Vt ventral.

different layers of the reticular wall are often very distinct: the tunica serosa appears as a thin echoic line on the outside and the tunica muscularis as a thin hypoechoic line in the middle, and the tunica mucosa combined with the tela submucosa on the inside are distinct. In contrast to reticuloperitonitis, there are no signs of inflammation, such as echoic fibrin deposits or abscesses. Furthermore, an anechoic seam of varying width is evident between the reticulum and spleen because the capillary space between these two organs is enlarged by the fluid.

Causes of Noninflammatory Ascites

The most common causes of noninflammatory ascites attributable to vascular congestion include chronic right-sided cardiac insufficiency, mediastinal masses, chronic liver and kidney diseases, small intestinal ileus and enteropathies, tumors of the peritoneum, and caudal vena cava thrombosis or compression (**Table 2**).

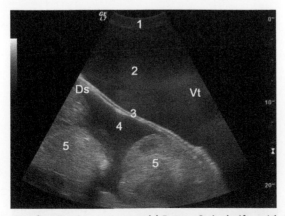

Fig. 4. Ultrasonogram of ascites in a 1.5-year-old Brown Swiss heifer with thrombosis of the caudal vena, imaged from the right flank. Loops of small intestine are displaced dorsally by hypoechoic ascites fluid. 1, lateral abdominal wall; 2, extraomental ascites fluid; 3, large omentum; 4 intraomental ascites fluid; 5 small intestine. Ds, dorsal; Vt, ventral. See also **Fig. 13**.

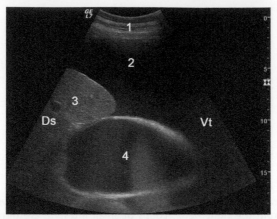

Fig. 5. Ultrasonogram of the liver and gallbladder of a cow with ascites, imaged from the 10th intercostal space on the right side. The liver and gallbladder are displaced medially by anechoic ascites fluid. 1, lateral abdominal wall; 2, ascites; 3, liver; 4, gallbladder. Ds, dorsal; Vt, ventral.

Right-Sided Cardiac Insufficiency as the Cause of Ascites

Ascites caused by right-sided cardiac insufficiency (traumatic pericarditis, valvular endocarditis, idiopathic cardiomyopathy, cardiac lymphosarcoma) is accompanied by abnormal auscultatory findings, such as tachycardia, pericardial or endocardial heart sounds, or cardiac arrhythmia (summation gallop heart sound in cardiomyopathy).[23] The jugular veins are distended; there is submandibular, presternal, and ventral edema. Pleural effusion, dilation of the caudal vena cava, and a change in its cross-sectional appearance from triangular to oval or circular are consistent and specific ultrasonographic findings of right-sided cardiac insufficiency.[2] The activities of liver enzymes are increased because of liver congestion.

Mediastinal Masses as the Cause of Ascites

Compression of the caudal vena cava by a mediastinal mass, such as an abscess or tumor, also results in a change in its cross-sectional shape to oval or circular, which

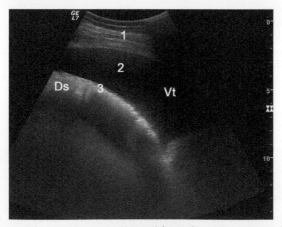

Fig. 6. Ultrasonogram of ascites in a cow, imaged from the 10th intercostal space on the left side. The rumen is displaced dorsomedially by anechoic ascites fluid. 1, lateral abdominal wall; 2, ascites fluid; 3, rumen. Ds, dorsal; Vt, ventral.

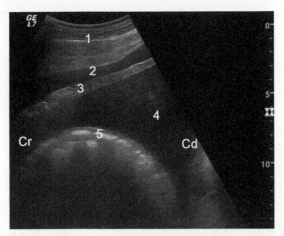

Fig. 7. Ultrasonogram of the reticular region of a cow with ascites, imaged from the sternal part of the ventral abdomen. The reticulum is displaced dorsally by hypoechoic ascites fluid. 1, ventral abdominal wall; 2, musculophrenic vein; 3, diaphragm; 4, ascites fluid; 5, reticulum. Cd, caudal; Cr, cranial.

can be detected sonographically in the 11th and 12th intercostal spaces. Jugular distension is not a feature of this condition.[2]

Liver Disease as the Cause of Ascites

Ascites is common in liver disease and occurs when hepatic perfusion is compromised by liver cirrhosis, fascioliasis, or a tumor or abscess causing intrahepatic congestion. Hypoalbuminemia from impaired albumin synthesis is responsible for a decrease in intravascular oncotic pressure in liver cirrhosis and fascioliasis.[2] In addition, an increase in pressure in the venous part of the splanchnic circulation because of impaired liver perfusion causes transudation of fluid into the peritoneal space. In cattle, severe hypoalbuminemia is always accompanied clinically by edema. Prehepatic portal hypertension caused by portal vein thrombosis alone in the absence of liver disease is not associated with ascites, which underlines the crucial role of decreased oncotic pressure in the pathogenesis of ascites[24]; the oncotic pressure remains unchanged because arterial perfusion compensates for lost venous perfusion. In addition to ascites, characteristic ultrasonographic features of portal hypertension include focal changes with abscesses or tumors, calcification of bile ducts with fascioliasis, and dilation of the portal vein. Blood analysis shows hypoalbuminemia and increased activity of liver enzymes, and microscopic examination of bile collected under ultrasound guidance shows common liver fluke ova.[25] Fascioliasis is commonly complicated by concurrent peritonitis, and analysis of peritoneal fluid may show a modified transudate or even an exudate with an elevated eosinophil count. The principal ultrasonographic finding in cows with hepatic fibrosis attributable to *Senecio alpinus* poisoning was severe noninflammatory ascites.[26] The liver parenchyma of all cows appeared heterogeneous and often had nodular changes; all cows had portal hypertension caused by intrahepatic changes, dilation of the portal vein, and a decrease in the diameter of the caudal vena cava lumen because of reduced liver perfusion. Portal hypertension also resulted in edema of the gall bladder wall, small intestines, and greater omentum. Cows with hepatocellular carcinoma had severe focal or diffuse hepatic changes but no ascites.[27,28]

Table 2
Noninflammatory ascites in cattle: causes and ultrasonographic, clinical, and laboratory findings

Affected Organ	Disease	Main Clinical and Laboratory Findings	Ultrasonographic Findings
Heart	Right-sided cardiac insufficiency	1. Abnormal auscultatory findings, such as tachycardia, murmur, dysrhythmia 2. Distension of jugular veins 3. Edema 4. Elevated activities of liver enzymes	1. Abnormal echocardiographic findings 2. Pleural effusion 3. Dilatation of caudal vena cava
Mediastinum	Mediastinal mass, such as a tumor or abscess	1. Radiodensity on thoracic radiograph 2. Elevated activities of liver enzymes	Dilatation of caudal vena cava
Liver	Liver cirrhosis Fascioliasis Liver abscess Liver tumor	1. Elevated activities of liver enzymes 2. Liver fluke eggs in feces or bile (fascioliasis) 3. Shorter-than-normal glutaraldehyde clotting test (liver abscess)	1. Dilatation of portal vein (liver cirrhosis) 2. Calcification of bile ducts (fascioliasis) 3. Discrete changes in liver parenchyma (abscess, tumor)
Kidneys	Nephrotic syndrome Amyloid nephrosis	1. Edema 2. Enlarged left kidney on rectal examination 3. Diarrhea 4. Massive proteinuria 5. Elevated level of serum urea	Enlargement of kidneys; renal parenchyma diffusely echogenic in amyloid nephrosis
Intestine	Volvulus Enteropathy	1. Signs of ileus (volvulus) 2. Weight loss, diarrhea (enteropathy)	Jejunum dilated and static
Peritoneum	Tumors, such as mesothelioma	No specific findings	1. Neoplastic changes of peritoneum, omentum, and serosal surfaces 2. Metastatic tumors in other organs (not in mesothelioma)
Blood vessels	Thrombosis of caudal vena cava	1. Metastatic suppurative bronchopneumonia 2. Epistaxis 3. Elevated activities of liver enzymes	1. Dilatation of caudal vena cava 2. Thrombus in caudal vena cava (sometimes)

Kidney Disease as the Cause of Ascites

Amyloid nephrosis is accompanied by massive protein loss in the urine resulting in hypoproteinemia, edema, and ascites.[29] The kidneys are enlarged, and affected cattle have diarrhea and weight loss. Ultrasonography confirms enlargement of the kidneys and shows diffuse parenchymal changes. The histologic examination of a biopsy specimen confirms the diagnosis.

Ileus as the Cause of Ascites

Various forms of ileus of the small and large intestines can cause ascites through transudation as a result of vascular constriction. Ileus of the small intestine includes all conditions that are accompanied by displacement, twisting, and constriction of the intestine, including volvulus, compression, invagination, incarceration, and obstruction.[30] Dilated, nonmotile loops of small intestine that may or may not be separated from each other by fluid is a typical ultrasonographic finding of ileus (**Fig. 8**). Occasionally it is possible to visualize the cause of the ileus, for instance, intestinal obstruction by blood coagula in hemorrhagic bowel syndrome (**Fig. 9**). Cecal torsion is the main disorder of the large intestine that causes transudation and peritoneal fluid accumulation (**Fig. 10**).[31,32] Ileus and cecal dilation are readily diagnosed clinically and sonographically and differentiated from other forms of ascites.[30–32]

Tumors of the Peritoneum, Serous Membranes, and Omentum

Tumors of the visceral and parietal peritoneum and omentum are rare in cattle. They are mostly multiple, firm, nodular, or pedunculated tumors or tumors with a broad attachment. Accompanying nonspecific clinical signs include weight loss, poor appetite, and ascites.[2] The tumors often can be palpated transrectally. These tumors include mesothelioma,[19,21,32] metastatic hepatic, gastrointestinal, urinary tract, or pulmonary carcinoma as well as lymphoma. The differential diagnosis of peritoneal changes palpated transrectally includes extrapulmonary tuberculosis of the serous membranes, and the differential diagnosis of palpable mesenteric changes includes fat necrosis. Cows with mesothelioma have severe ascites.[19–21,32] Ultrasonographically, the tumors appear as uneven nodular masses on the peritoneum and serosal

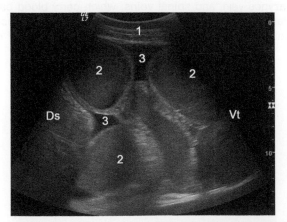

Fig. 8. Ultrasonogram of the abdomen of a cow with ileus because of intussusception, imaged from the 12th intercostal space on the right side. There is accumulation of anechoic fluid (transudate) and dilated loops of small intestine. 1, abdominal wall; 2, dilated loops of small intestine; 3, anechoic fluid between the loops of small intestine. Ds, dorsal; Vt, ventral.

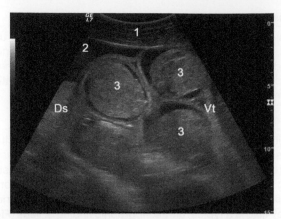

Fig. 9. Ultrasonogram of the abdomen of a cow with hemorrhagic bowel syndrome, imaged from the right flank. Anechoic fluid (transudate) and dilated loops of small intestine. Small intestine contains echoic material surrounded by an anechoic rim consistent with a blood clot. 1, abdominal wall; 2, anechoic fluid between loops of small intestine; 3, small intestine with a blood clot. Ds, dorsal; Vt, ventral.

surface of abdominal organs, such as the rumen, omasum, or spleen (**Fig. 11**). The greater omentum, suspended in ascites fluid, may also be affected by nodular changes (**Fig. 12**). The aspirated peritoneal fluid is a modified transudate with a dark yellow to red color and may have a high erythrocyte count. The cytologic diagnosis of mesothelioma is often limited by the paucity of cells in the aspirated fluid. The final diagnosis is based on histologic, immunohistologic, or electron microscopic examination of the tumor.

Obstruction and Compression of the Caudal Vena Cava as the Cause of Ascites

Thrombosis and compression of the caudal vena cava by an abscess or tumor can lead to ascites. Although white thrombi of the caudal vena cava are relatively common, they are a rare cause of ascites because of the collateral circulation through the milk veins, azygos vein, and spinal veins, which carry blood back to the heart when the caudal vena cava is obstructed. However, ascites occurs when the thrombus is located cranial to the liver and occupies at least half of the lumen of

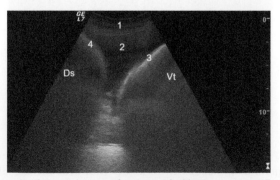

Fig. 10. Ultrasonogram of the abdomen of a cow with dilation and retroflexion of the cecum, imaged from the right flank. The cecum and colon are separated by anechoic fluid (transudate). 1, lateral abdominal wall; 2, fluid accumulation; 3, cecum; 4, colon. Ds, dorsal; Vt, ventral.

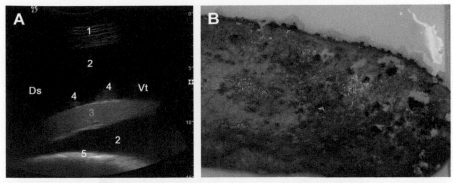

Fig. 11. Ultrasonogram (*A*) and postmortem view (*B*) of the spleen of a cow with mesothelioma, imaged from the 10th intercostal space on the left side. The spleen is covered with yellow tumorous nodules identified histologically as mesothelioma. 1, lateral abdominal wall; 2, ascites; 3, spleen; 4, tumorous alterations of the spleen (mesothelioma); 5, rumen. Ds, dorsal; Vt, ventral.

the vessel[33,34] or when both milk veins are thrombosed after the infusion of irritating solutions and no longer contribute to the collateral circulation.[35] Caudal vena cava thrombosis may cause ascites in young cattle[36] and bulls because of the small diameter and capacity of the milk vein (**Fig. 13**). Obstruction or compression of the caudal vena cava leads to congestion of the vessel, which increases its diameter and changes its cross-sectional shape from triangular to oval or circular. This congestion is best visualized in the liver region at the 11th and 12th intercostal spaces on the right side (**Fig. 14**).[35–39] As a result of liver congestion, the veins joining the congested vena cava, particularly the right hepatic vein, appear as prominent and markedly dilated vessels (**Fig. 15**), the liver has an obtuse marginal angle, and the wall of the gall bladder is edematous (**Fig. 16**). The thrombus rarely can be visualized

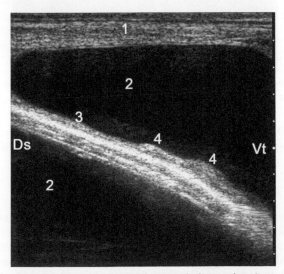

Fig. 12. Ultrasonogram of ascites in a cow with mesothelioma showing nodular changes of the greater omentum, imaged from the right flank. 1, lateral abdominal wall; 2, ascites; 3, greater omentum; 4, tumorous nodules (mesothelioma). Ds, dorsal; Vt, ventral.

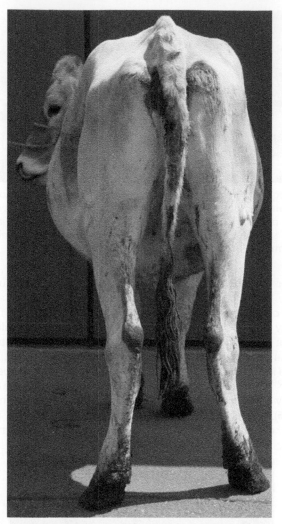

Fig. 13. Pear-shaped abdomen in a Brown Swiss heifer with ascites as a sequel of thrombosis of the caudal vena cava. See also **Fig. 4.**

sonographically (**Fig. 17**) because usually it is in a section of the vena cava superimposed by the lungs.[38] Likewise, thrombi in the tributaries of the vena cava are rarely visualized.[40]

INFLAMMATORY ASCITES (PERITONITIS)

Inflammatory ascites is associated with peritonitis, which is defined as peritoneal inflammation resulting from trauma and/or bacterial infection.[2] Peritonitis is often parasite related and in rare cases caused by medications. Peritonitis is characterized by peritoneal alteration and proliferation as well as exudation and can be focal or diffuse and acute or chronic. Bacteria commonly involved in the cause of peritonitis include *Trueperella pyogenes*, streptococci, staphylococci, and *Escherichia coli*, which are introduced directly into the peritoneal cavity via perforating wounds

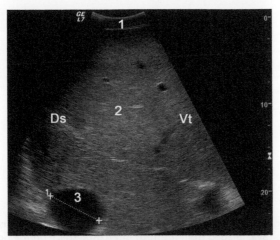

Fig. 14. Ultrasonogram of the liver in a cow with thrombosis of the caudal vena cava, imaged from the 11th intercostal space on the right side. The caudal vena cava, which normally is triangular in cross section, has become oval in cross section because of congestion and dilation. 1, lateral abdominal wall; 2, liver; 3, dilated caudal vena cava with oval cross section and a large diameter of 6.24 cm. Ds, dorsal; Vt, ventral.

or indirectly via the hematogenous or lymphatic route. A perforating reticular foreign body is the most common cause of peritonitis (**Table 3**). Perforating abomasal ulcer is also a common cause of peritonitis in postpartum dairy cows, whereas perforating injuries of the uterus, cervix, vagina, bladder, small and large intestines, or rectum associated with parturition, urolithiasis, or transrectal examination are less common. Peritonitis may also occur after laparotomy[41] or as a sequel to ulcerative colitis and proctitis.[42] Migrating juvenile stages of *Fasciola hepatica* occasionally cause peritonitis, whereas rupture of an intraperitoneal abscess is a rare cause. A

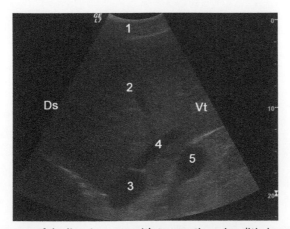

Fig. 15. Ultrasonogram of the liver in a cow with traumatic pericarditis, imaged from the 11th intercostal space on the right side. The caudal vena cava and right hepatic vein are dilated. 1, lateral abdominal wall; 2, liver; 3, dilated caudal vena cava with oval cross section; 4, dilated right hepatic vein; 5, portal vein. Ds, dorsal; Vt, ventral.

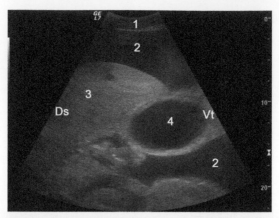

Fig. 16. Ultrasonogram of the liver in a Brown Swiss heifer with ascites caused by thrombosis of the caudal vena cava, imaged from the 10th intercostal space on the right side. The liver has an obtuse marginal angle and the wall of the gallbladder is edematous. 1, abdominal wall; 2, ascites fluid; 3, liver; 4, gallbladder. Ds, dorsal; Vt, ventral. See also **Figs. 4** and **13**.

tentative diagnosis of peritonitis is usually straightforward after a perforating injury of the abdominal wall associated with ruminal trocarization,[41] horn injury, or after laparotomy.

Ultrasonographic Findings of Focal and Generalized Peritonitis

The localization, extent, and type of changes caused by peritonitis vary greatly depending on the severity and cause of peritonitis. Exudation may be absent in fibrinous peritonitis, and the only lesions seen sonographically may be changes on the organ surface and/or peritoneum. These changes are typical of traumatic reticuloperitonitis and perforating abomasal ulcer, in which an uneven organ surface with echoic deposits (**Fig. 18**), often containing fluid inclusions (**Fig. 19**) and surrounded by fluid (**Fig. 20**), is seen instead of the normal smooth surface. The extent of the

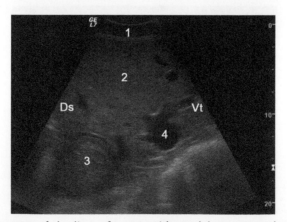

Fig. 17. Ultrasonogram of the liver of a cow with caudal vena cava thrombosis, imaged from the 11th intercostal space on the right side. The caudal vena cava is occupied by an echoic thrombus. 1, abdominal wall; 2, liver; 3, echoic thrombus in the caudal vena cava; 4, portal vein. Ds, dorsal; Vt, ventral.

Table 3
Causes of peritonitis in cattle

Organ	Cause	Nature of Disease
Reticulum	Foreign body	Localized or generalized peritonitis
Abomasum	Type-3 abomasal ulcer	Localized peritonitis
	Type-4 abomasal ulcer	Generalized peritonitis
Small/large intestine	Ileus	Generalized peritonitis
	Intestinal ulcer	Generalized peritonitis
	Intestinal tumor	Generalized peritonitis
	Migrating *Fasciola hepatica* larvae	Fibrinous peritonitis
Rectum	Injury during rectal palpation	Localized or generalized peritonitis
Uterus	Injury during parturition	Localized or generalized peritonitis
	Injury during intrauterine infusion	Localized or generalized peritonitis
Vagina	Sadism	Localized or generalized peritonitis
Urinary bladder	Injury during catheterization (females)	Localized or generalized peritonitis, and uroperitoneum after rupture
	Rupture caused by obstructive urolithiasis (males)	of urinary bladder
Abdominal wall	Trocarization of rumen	Localized or generalized peritonitis,
	Laparotomy	involving ingesta after trocarization
	Perforating injury (eg, injury caused by horns)	of rumen
All abdominal organs	Rupture of abscess	Localized or generalized peritonitis
Systemic infection	Pasteurellosis, tuberculosis, anthrax	Generalized peritonitis

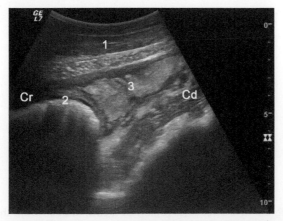

Fig. 18. Ultrasonogram of the reticulum in a cow with traumatic reticuloperitonitis, imaged from the sternal part of the abdomen. There are massive fibrin deposits caudal to the reticulum. 1, abdominal wall; 2, reticulum; 3, echoic fibrin deposits. Cd, caudal; Cr cranial.

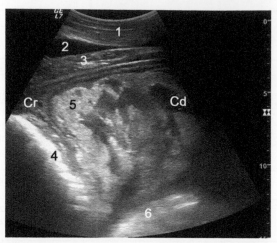

Fig. 19. Ultrasonogram of the reticular region in a cow with traumatic reticuloperitonitis, imaged from the sternal part of the abdomen. There are massive fibrin deposits and some fluid pockets between the reticulum and the rumen. 1, abdominal wall; 2, musculophrenic vein; 3, diaphragm; 4, reticulum; 5, echoic deposits with fluid pockets; 6, anterior dorsal blind sac of the rumen. Cd, caudal; Cr, cranial.

inflammatory exudation varies greatly and is usually limited to small effusions in the caudoventral region of the reticulum in cattle with hardware disease. In these cases, the reticulum, the dorsal blind sac of the rumen, and sometimes the cranial part of the ventral sac of the rumen are displaced dorsally by the effusion. Generalized peritonitis may be accompanied by massive fluid accumulation, which surrounds the organs and displaces them dorsally. Depending on the cell count and amount of fibrin, the fluid may appear anechoic (**Fig. 21**), hypoechoic (**Fig. 22**), or echoic (**Fig. 23**). Fibrin septa that form fluid compartments (**Fig. 24**) and floating fibrin strands are often seen running in a spiderweblike fashion between organs or between an organ and the parietal peritoneum. Often the fluid appears chambered in a

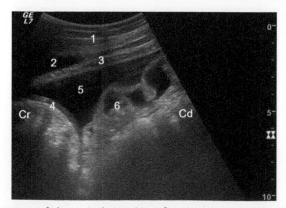

Fig. 20. Ultrasonogram of the reticular region of a cow, imaged from the sternal part of the abdomen. An effusion and fibrin deposits are evident caudal to the reticulum. 1, abdominal wall; 2, musculophrenic vein; 3, diaphragm; 4, reticulum; 5, effusion; 6, fibrin deposits. Cd, caudal; Cr, cranial.

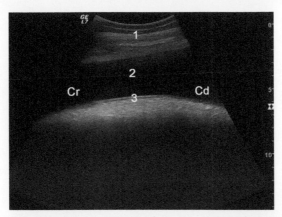

Fig. 21. Ultrasonogram of ascites in a cow with type 4 abomasal ulcer, imaged from the ventral part of the right abdomen. The ascites fluid is anechoic. 1, ventral abdominal wall; 2, ascites fluid; 3, rumen. Cd, caudal; Cr, cranial.

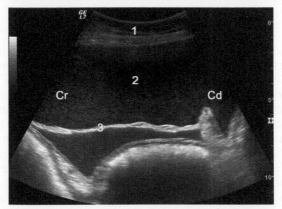

Fig. 22. Ultrasonogram of ascites in a cow with generalized peritonitis, imaged from the ventral abdominal wall. The ascites fluid is hypoechoic. 1, ventral abdominal wall; 2, hypoechoic ascites fluid; 3, fibrin strand. Cd, caudal; Cr, cranial.

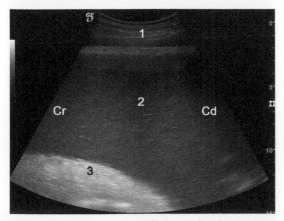

Fig. 23. Ultrasonogram of ascites in a cow with generalized peritonitis, imaged from the ventral abdominal wall. The ascites fluid is echoic. 1, ventral abdominal wall; 2, echoic ascites fluid; 3, fibrin deposits. Cd, caudal; Cr, cranial.

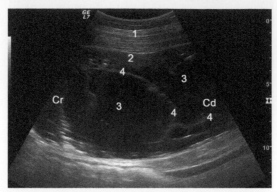

Fig. 24. Ultrasonogram of ascites in a cow with generalized peritonitis caused by type 4 abomasal ulcer, imaged from the ventral abdominal wall. The hypoechoic ascites fluid is separated by strands of fibrin. 1, ventral abdominal wall; 2, sediment on the floor of the abdomen; 3, fluid accumulation; 4, strands of fibrin. Cd, caudal; Cr, cranial.

spongelike fashion by strands of fibrin (**Figs. 25** and **26**). A layer of sediment composed of echoic cells and fibrin and an anechoic supernatant may be seen when there are many cells and fibrin (see **Fig. 24**), or abdominal organs may be coated with fibrinous deposits (**Fig. 27**) that contain gaseous inclusions of microbial origin (**Fig. 28**). When gastrointestinal contents escape into the peritoneal cavity, for instance, after abomasal or intestinal rupture, echoic ingesta may be seen coating some of the organs. The intestinal walls are often thickened, and echoic fibrin and inflammatory fluid are seen between loops of intestines in cattle with generalized peritonitis. Intestinal motility is usually severely reduced or absent because of adhesions, and diarrhea is common. However, based on ultrasonographic appearance alone, it is often not possible to differentiate a transudate, a modified transudate of noninflammatory ascites, and an exudate; the analysis of fluid collected by abdominocentesis is required for a diagnosis.

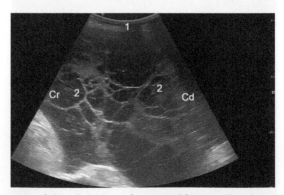

Fig. 25. Ultrasonogram of the abdomen of a cow with generalized peritonitis caused by a perforating foreign body in the abomasum, imaged from the ventral abdominal wall. The peritoneal fluid is separated into chambers by strands of fibrin, giving it a spongelike appearance. 1, ventral abdominal wall; 2, multi-chambered fibrin network. Cd, caudal; Cr cranial.

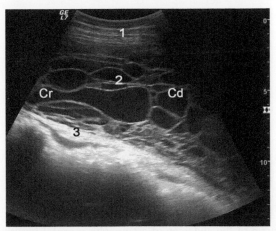

Fig. 26. Ultrasonogram of the abdomen of a cow with generalized peritonitis caused by perforation of the uterus, imaged from the ventral abdominal wall. The peritoneal fluid is separated into chambers by strands of fibrin, giving it a spongelike appearance. 1, ventral abdominal wall; 2, multi-chambered fibrin network; 3, greater omentum. Cd, caudal; Cr cranial.

Omental Bursitis

Omental bursitis is a special form of peritonitis characterized by the accumulation of watery, putrid, foul-smelling exudate in the omental bursa. Peritonitis is limited to the bursa and demarcated from the remaining abdominal cavity by a capsule of varying thickness. Reticular foreign bodies, ruminal perforation or ulcers, abomasal ulcers, and laparotomies are the most common causes.[43] Ultrasonographically, purulent omental bursitis appears as fluid accumulation of varying but often considerable size between the abdominal wall and the ventral sac of the rumen (**Fig. 29**). Extreme cases involve the entire ruminal width and length, extending from the naval to the

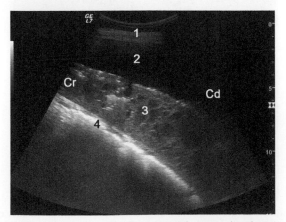

Fig. 27. Ultrasonogram of the abdomen of a cow with generalized peritonitis caused by a perforating reticular foreign body, imaged from the ventral abdominal wall. A thick fibrin layer covers the ventral sac of the rumen. 1, ventral abdominal wall; 2, anechoic fluid; 3, fibrin deposits on the ventral aspect of the ruminal wall; 4, rumen. Cd, caudal; Cr, cranial.

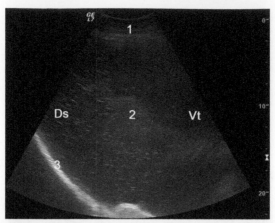

Fig. 28. Ultrasonogram of the abdomen of a cow with omental bursitis caused by type 4 abomasal ulcer, imaged from the 10th intercostal space on the left side. The fluid in the omental bursa is characterized by echoic stippling indicating microbial gas production. 1, lateral abdominal wall; 2, fluid in the omental bursa with echoic stippling; 3, ruminal wall. Ds, dorsal; Vt, ventral.

udder, and measure more than 10 cm vertically. The ultrasonographic appearance of the fluid and the fibrin deposits vary, and the echoic leaves of the bursa sometimes can be seen. A characteristic difference between omental bursitis and generalized peritonitis is that the former is restricted to the region ventral and lateral to the rumen on the left side, whereas the latter also involves the right side of the abdomen. Furthermore, the general demeanor and appetite are more severely affected in cattle with generalized peritonitis.

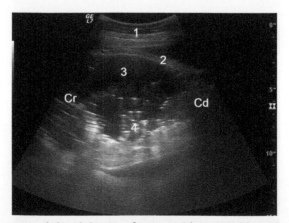

Fig. 29. Ultrasonogram of the abdomen of a cow with omental bursitis caused by type 4 abomasal ulcer, imaged from the ventral abdominal wall. There is echoic stippling of the fluid in the omental bursa indicating microbial gas production. 1, ventral abdominal wall; 2, greater omentum; 3, fluid in the omental bursa with echoic stippling; 4, gas inclusions. Cd, caudal; Cr, cranial.

UROPERITONEUM

Uroperitoneum is accumulation of urine in the peritoneal cavity. A review of the causes, diagnosis, and treatment of uroperitoneum in cattle was recently published.[44] Uroperitoneum can result from leakage of urine from the kidneys, ureters, urinary bladder, and urethra[45] as well as from rupture of a persistent urachus.[46]

The most common cause of bladder rupture is dystocia in cows[23,47–50] and urinary obstruction[49] associated with urolithiasis or urethral compression by a hematoma[51] in male cattle. A persistent urachus may rupture spontaneously for reasons that remain unclear. This rupture has been described in calves[52,53] and in young[54] and mature cattle.[46,55] The main clinical sign is pear-shaped enlargement of the abdomen.

Ultrasonography shows massive fluid accumulation involving the entire abdomen and dorsally displaced abdominal organs that are suspended in the fluid. The site of bladder rupture can sometimes be detected during transrectal sonographic examination. The ruptured bladder may be collapsed and flaccid and contain little or no urine or contain moderate amounts of urine when the defect is sealed by fibrin.[56] When a persistent urachus exerts traction on the bladder, the urine-filled transition from the bladder to the urachus can be seen sonographically (**Fig. 30**). Sometimes the bladder is surrounded by urine. A completely empty bladder may not be seen.

The diagnosis is confirmed by abdominocentesis and analysis of the aspirated fluid. The fluid is light yellow or colorless and occasionally smells of urine. Comparison of urea and creatinine concentrations of the aspirated fluid and blood reliably differentiates urine and a transudate. With uroperitoneum, both variables are much higher in the aspirated fluid than in blood; a peritoneal fluid-to-serum creatinine concentration ratio of 2 or greater is diagnostic of uroperitoneum.[23]

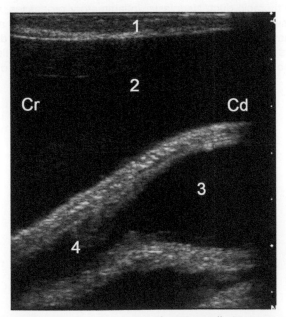

Fig. 30. Ultrasonogram of the bladder obtained transrectally in a cow with rupture of a persistent urachus. The persistent urachus is visible at the cranial pole of the bladder. 1, rectum; 2, anechoic fluid (uroperitoneum) surrounding the bladder; 3, bladder; 4, persistent urachus. Cd, caudal; Cr, cranial.

A flexible endoscope is used to differentiate bladder rupture and urachal rupture.[46] With urachal rupture, the bladder is stretched longitudinally and the endoscope can be introduced into the urine-filled urachus.[46]

HEMOPERITONEUM

Hemoperitoneum is the presence of blood in the peritoneal cavity. It is accompanied clinically by pronounced anemia and decreased hematocrit. It is rare in cattle and always results from hemorrhage from a ruptured blood vessel or spleen or is related to a clotting disorder.[2] The ultrasonographic appearance of the fluid varies from hypoechoic to hyperechoic depending on the degree of clotting. A symptomatic diagnosis is made when abdominocentesis produces a hemorrhagic aspirate, but the measurement of clotting factors or a laparotomy may be required for an etiologic diagnosis. There have been 2 reports of hemoperitoneum in cattle as a result of a ruptured metastatic granulosa cell tumor[57,58] and another because of rupture of the gall bladder.[59] All animals had marked anemia and the abdominal fluid was anechoic. One of the cows with metastatic granulosa cell tumor had multiple metastatic tumors in the abdominal cavity that appeared ultrasonographically as multi-chambered spongelike structures of varying size (**Figs. 31** and **32**). Hemorrhage was caused by rupture of the cystic tumor capsule. Two other (Braun, unpublished, 2010) cases referred to the author's clinic concerned 2 cows with hemoperitoneum following transrectal manual rupture of an ovarian cyst and enucleation of a corpus luteum. In both cases, the peritoneal fluid was hypoechoic.

CHYLOUS ASCITES

Chylous ascites is the accumulation of chyle in the peritoneal cavity and arises from a blockage of the thoracic duct. Neoplasia, inflammatory processes, tuberculosis, or trauma are causes of chylous ascites in people; but some cases are idiopathic.[60] This condition may also result from iatrogenic injury to lymph vessels during surgery.[61] The fluid appears hyperechoic; aspiration of viscous, milky, opaque fluid rich in triglycerides is diagnostic. Chylothorax and chyloperitoneum in a calf diagnosed using

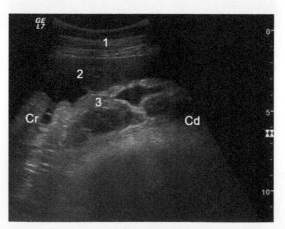

Fig. 31. Ultrasonogram of the abdomen of a cow with hemoabdomen caused by rupture of the capsule of a granulosa cell tumor, imaged from the right flank. Metastatic tumors are seen on the surface of internal organs. 1, abdominal wall; 2, anechoic fluid; 3, metastatic tumors. Cd, caudal; Cr, cranial.

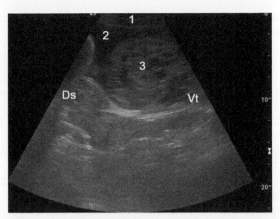

Fig. 32. Ultrasonogram of the abdomen of a cow with hemoabdomen caused by rupture of the capsule of a granulosa cell tumor, imaged from the right abdominal wall. Metastatic tumors are seen on the surface of internal organs. 1, ventral abdominal wall; 2, anechoic fluid; 3, metastatic tumors. Ds, dorsal; Vt, ventral.

mesenteric lymphangiography is the only published case in cattle.[62] Another case of chylothorax occurred in a 2-day-old calf as a result of thoracic vertebral fracture during birth.[63]

BILIARY ASCITES (BILE PERITONITIS)

Biliary ascites (bile peritonitis) is the term used to describe peritonitis caused by bile in the peritoneal cavity. Possible causes are perforation of the gall bladder by trauma or because of cholecystitis or iatrogenic rupture during procedures, such as aspiration of bile from the gall bladder. Only 3 cases of bile peritonitis have been reported in cattle, and all were the result of bile duct obstruction by concrement related to *Fasciola hepatica* infestation.[59] Typical clinical signs of cholestasis, including icterus and bilirubinuria, were seen in only one cow. Another cow had severe anemia because gall bladder rupture was accompanied by hemoperitoneum. Increased activity of the bile duct enzyme γ-glutamyl transferase and increased concentration of bilirubin are the main serum biochemical findings. Ultrasonographic examination of cows with gall bladder rupture shows biliary ascites, fibrin deposits on various organs, and strands of fibrin in the peritoneal cavity. In addition, there are fascioliasis-related changes in the liver, which primarily include calcified echoic bile ducts with distal acoustic shadowing and cholestasis. The appearance of the aspirated fluid varied widely in the 3 cows seen at the author's clinic and was hemorrhagic, bilious, and greenish opaque and fibrinous, respectively. In one cow, the gall bladder contained sediment and had a thickened wall and irregular contour, which was related to the rupture. The bilirubin concentration is increased in bile-containing ascites fluid[64] and should be measured when the assessment of the aspirated fluid is not straightforward. A bilirubin concentration greater than 8.5 μmol/L indicates rupture of the gall bladder.[65]

DIFFERENTIAL DIAGNOSIS OF INTRA-ABDOMINAL FLUID ACCUMULATION

The differential diagnosis of intra-abdominal fluid accumulation includes normal pregnancy and hydrops allantois. However, the diagnosis of pregnancy and hydrops is usually straightforward based on the results of transrectal examination. On sonograms, the uterine wall is seen as a thick echoic line and the caruncles appear as fist-sized structures attached to the uterine wall. Furthermore, fetal parts are seen in pregnant cows, and a heartbeat is often detected in live fetuses.

REFERENCES

1. Schreiber MA, Kremer H. Peritonealhöhle, Aszites und Bauchdecken. In: Kremer H, Dobrinski W, editors. Sonographische Diagnostik. Innere Medizin und angrenzende Gebiete. München (Germany); Wien (Austria); Baltimore (MD): Urban & Schwarzenberg; 1994. p. 235–41.
2. Braun U. Atlas und Lehrbuch der Ultraschalldiagnostik beim Rind. Berlin: Parey Buchverlag; 1997.
3. Braun U, Rauch S. Ultrasonographic evaluation of reticular motility during rest, eating, rumination and stress in 30 healthy cows. Vet Rec 2008;163(19):571–4.
4. Braun U, Schweizer A, Trösch L. Ultrasonography of the rumen of dairy cows. BMC Vet Res 2013;9:44.
5. Braun U, Blessing S. Ultrasonographic examination of the omasum in 30 healthy cows. Vet Rec 2006;159(24):812–5.
6. Braun U, Wild K, Guscetti F. Ultrasonographic examination of the abomasum of 50 cows. Vet Rec 1997;140(4):93–8.
7. Braun U, Marmier O. Ultrasonographic examination of the small intestine of cows. Vet Rec 1995;136(10):239–44.
8. Braun U, Amrein E. Ultrasonographic examination of the caecum and proximal and spiral ansa of the colon of cattle. Vet Rec 2001;149(2):45–8.
9. Braun U, Gerber D. Influence of age, breed, and stage of pregnancy on hepatic ultrasonographic findings in cows. Am J Vet Res 1994;55(9):1201–5.
10. Braun U, Sicher D. Ultrasonography of the spleen in 50 healthy cows. Vet J 2006; 171(3):513–8.
11. Braun U. Ultrasonographic examination of the right kidney in cows. Am J Vet Res 1991;52(12):1933–9.
12. Braun U. Ultrasonographic examination of the left kidney, the urinary bladder, and the urethra in cows. Zentralbl Veterinärmed A 1993;40(1):1–9.
13. Hirsch VM, Townsend HGG. Peritoneal fluid analysis in the diagnosis of abdominal disorders in cattle: a retrospective study. Can Vet J 1982;23(12):348–54.
14. Wilson AD, Hirsch VM, Osborne AD. Abdominocentesis in cattle: technique and criteria for diagnosis of peritonitis. Can Vet J 1985;26(2):74–80.
15. Kopcha M, Schultze AE. Peritoneal fluid. Part 1. Pathophysiology and classification of nonneoplastic effusions. Compend Contin Educ Pract Vet 1991;13(3):519–25.
16. Kopcha M, Schultze AE. Peritoneal fluid. Part 2. Abdominocentesis in cattle and interpretation of nonneoplastic samples. Compend Contin Educ Pract Vet 1991; 13(4):703–9.
17. Wittek T, Grosche A, Locher L, et al. Biochemical constituents of peritoneal fluid in cows. Vet Rec 2010;166(1):15–9.
18. Wittek T, Grosche A, Locher LF, et al. Diagnostic accuracy of d-dimer and other peritoneal fluid analysis measurements in dairy cows with peritonitis. J Vet Intern Med 2010;24:1211–7.
19. Wolfe DF, Carson RL, Hudson RS, et al. Mesothelioma in cattle: eight cases (1970-1988). J Am Vet Med Assoc 1991;199(4):486–91.
20. Milne MH, Mellor DJ, Barrett DC, et al. Observations on ascites in nine cattle. Vet Rec 2001;148(11):341–4.
21. Braun U, Gerspach C, Metzger L, et al. Ultrasonographic findings in a cow with ascites due to a mesothelioma. Vet Rec 2004;154(9):272–4.

22. Braun U, Rütten M, Bleul U, et al. Biphasisches Mesotheliom bei einer Braunvieh-kuh: Klinische, histomorphologische, immunhistochemische und elektronenmik-roskopische Befunde. Schweiz Arch Tierheilkd 2012;154(1):33–8.
23. Radostits OM, Gay CC, Hinchliff KW, et al. Veterinary Medicine. A Textbook of the Diseases of Cattle, Horses, Sheep, Pigs, and Goats. Edinburgh (Scotland): Saunders Elsevier; 2007. p. 562–3.
24. Matern S. Leber. In: Siegenthaler W, editor. Klinische Pathophysiologie. 6th edition. Stuttgart (Germany); New York: Georg Thieme; 1987. p. 864–900.
25. Braun U, Gerber D. Percutaneous ultrasound-guided cholecystocentesis in cows. Am J Vet Res 1992;53(7):1079–84.
26. Braun U, Linggi T, Pospischil A. Ultrasonographic findings in three cows with chronic ragwort (Senecio alpinus) poisoning. Vet Rec 1999;144(5):122–6.
27. Braun U, Caplazi P, Linggi T, et al. Polyglobulie infolge Leberkarzinom bei Rind und Schaf. Schweiz Arch Tierheilkd 1997;139(4):165–71.
28. Braun U, Nuss K, Soldati G, et al. Clinical and ultrasonographic findings in four cows with liver tumours. Vet Rec 2005;157(16):482–4.
29. Elitok UM, Elitok B, Unver O. Renal amyloidosis in cattle with inflammatory diseases. J Vet Intern Med 2008;22(2):450–5.
30. Braun U. Ultrasonography of the gastrointestinal tract in cattle. Vet Clin North Am Food Anim Pract 2009;25(3):567–90.
31. Braun U, Amrein E, Koller U, et al. Ultrasonographic findings in cows with dilatation, torsion and retroflexion of the caecum. Vet Rec 2002;150(3):75–9.
32. Braun U, Beckmann C, Gerspach C, et al. Clinical findings and treatment in cattle with caecal dilatation. BMC Vet Res 2012;8:75.
33. Adams OR. Hepatic changes resulting from partial ligation of the posterior vena cava in cattle. Am J Vet Res 1963;24(5):557–64.
34. Selman IE, Wiseman A, Petrie L, et al. A respiratory syndrome in cattle resulting from thrombosis of the posterior vena cava. Vet Rec 1974;94(20):459–66.
35. Braun U, Schefer U, Gerber D, et al. Ultrasonographic findings in a cow with ascites due to thrombosis of the caudal vena cava. Schweiz Arch Tierheilkd 1992;134(5):235–41.
36. Braun U, Schweizer G, Wehbrink D, et al. Ultraschallbefunde bei einem Rind mit Aszites infolge Thrombose der Vena cava caudalis. Tierärztl Prax 2005;33(G):389–94.
37. Braun U, Flückiger M, Feige K, et al. Diagnosis by ultrasonography of congestion of the caudal vena cava secondary to thrombosis in 12 cows. Vet Rec 2002;150(7):209–13.
38. Braun U, Salis F, Gerspach C. Sonographischer Nachweis eines echogenen Thrombus in der Vena cava caudalis bei einer Kuh. Schweiz Arch Tierheilkd 2003;145(7):340–1.
39. Braun U, Feller B, Trachsel D, et al. Lungenabszess, Pleuraerguss und Aszites bei einem Rind mit Vena-cava-caudalis-Thrombose. Dtsch Tierärztl Wochenschr 2007;114(5):165–70.
40. Mohamed T, Sato H, Kurosawa T, et al. Ultrasonographic localisation of thrombi in the caudal vena cava and hepatic veins in a heifer. Vet J 2004;168(1):103–6.
41. Braun U, Pusterla N, Anliker H. Ultrasonographic findings in three cows with peritonitis in the left flank region. Vet Rec 1998;142(13):338–40.
42. Braun U, Hilbe M, Gerspach C, et al. Ulzerierende Colitis und Proktitis bei zwei Braunviehkühen. Schweiz Arch Tierheilkd 2015;157:204–8.
43. Dirksen G. Bauchhöhlenabszesse, Netzbeutelentzündung. In: Dirksen G, Gründer HD, Stöber M, editors. Innere Medizin und Chirurgie des Rindes. Berlin: Parey Buchverlag; 2002. p. 671–4.

44. Braun U, Nuss K. Uroperitoneum in cattle: Ultrasonographic findings, diagnosis and treatment. Acta Vet Scand 2015;57:36.
45. Maxie MG, Newman SJ. Acquired anatomic variations. In: Maxie MG, editor. Jubb, Kennedy, and Palmer's Pathology of Domestic Animals, vol. 2, 5th edition. Edinburgh (Scotland): Saunders Elsevier; 2007. p. 506–7.
46. Braun U, Previtali M, Fürst A, et al. Zystoskopie bei einem Rind mit Urachus persistens-Ruptur. Schweiz Arch Tierheilkd 2009;151(11):539–44.
47. Smith JA, Divers TJ, Lamp TM. Ruptured urinary bladder in a post-parturient cow. Cornell Vet 1983;73(1):3–12.
48. Carr EA, Schott HC, Barrington GM, et al. Ruptured urinary bladder after dystocia in a cow. J Am Vet Med Assoc 1993;202(4):631–2.
49. Gründer HD. Krankheiten von Harnleiter, Harnblase und Harnröhre. In: Dirksen G, Gründer HD, Stöber M, editors. Innere Medizin und Chirurgie des Rindes. Berlin: Parey Buchverlag; 2002. p. 719–36.
50. Braun U, Wetli U, Bryce B, et al. Clinical, ultrasonographic and endoscopic findings in a cow with bladder rupture caused by suppurative necrotising cystitis. Vet Rec 2007;161(20):700–2.
51. Braun U, Trösch L, Sydler T. Ruptured urinary bladder attributable to urethral compression by a haematoma after vertebral fracture in a bull. Acta Vet Scand 2014;56:17.
52. Bell GJC, Macrae AI, Milne EM, et al. Extensive uroperitoneum and pleural effusion associated with necrotic urachal remnant in a bull calf. Vet Rec 2004; 154(16):508–9.
53. Nikahval B, Khafi MSA. Congenital persistent urachus, urethral obstruction and uroperitoneum in a calf. Iran J Vet Res 2013;14(2):158–60.
54. Baxter GM, Zamos DT, Mueller POE. Uroperitoneum attributable to ruptured urachus in a yearling bull. J Am Vet Med Assoc 1992;200(4):517–20.
55. Marques LC, Marques JA, Marques ICS, et al. Dilatação cística do úraco europeritônio em touros: relato de cinco casos. Arq Bras Med Vet Zootec 2010;62(6): 1320–4.
56. Floeck M. Ultrasonography of bovine urinary tract disorders. Vet Clin North Am Food Anim Pract 2009;25(3):651–67.
57. Masseau I, Fecteau G, Desrochers A, et al. Hemoperitoneum caused by the rupture of a granulosa cell tumor in a Holstein heifer. Can Vet J 2004;45(6): 504–6.
58. Trösch L, Müller K, Brosinski K, et al. Hämoabdomen und Hämothorax bei einem Rind mit metastasierendem Granulosazelltumor. Schweiz Arch Tierheilkd 2015; 157(6):345–7.
59. Braun U, Schweizer G, Pospischil A. Clinical and ultrasonographic findings in three cows with ruptured gallbladders. Vet Rec 2005;156(11):351–3.
60. Siegenthaler W. Allgemeine Differenzialdiagnose des Ikterus. In: Siegenthaler W, editor. Siegenthalers Differenzialdiagnose. Innere Krankheiten – vom Symptom zur Diagnose. Stuttgart (Germany): Georg Thieme Verlag; 2000. p. 773–809.
61. Lee EW, Shin JH, Ko HK, et al. Lymphangiography to treat postoperative lymphatic leakage: a technical review. Korean J Radiol 2014;15(6):724–32.
62. Cruz AM, Riley CB, MacDonald DG, et al. Use of mesenteric lymphangiography in a calf with chylothorax and chyloperitoneum. J Am Vet Med Assoc 1995; 206(10):1567–71.
63. Pusterla N, Pusterla JB, Thür B, et al. Chylothorax bei einem Kalb. Tierärztl Prax 1996;24(6):554–8.

64. Argyres MI, Porter J, Rizeq MN. Diagnosis of clinically unsuspected gallbladder rupture by peritoneal fluid cytology - a case report. Acta Cytol 1998;42(4):973–7.
65. Dirksen G. Normalbefunde und wichtigste Abweichungen des Bauchhöhlenpunktates beim Rind. In: Dirksen G, Gründer HD, Stöber M, editors. Die klinische Untersuchung des Rindes. Berlin: Paul Parey; 1990. p. 392–3.

Ultrasonographic Examination of the Reticulum, Rumen, Omasum, Abomasum, and Liver in Calves

Ueli Braun, Prof Dr Med Vet, Dr Med Vet H C

KEYWORDS

- Cattle • Calf • Ultrasonography • Reticulum • Rumen • Abomasum
- Esophageal groove reflex • Ruminal drinker

KEY POINTS

- Abdominal ultrasonography is primarily indicated for the assessment of the gastrointestinal tract of diseased calves but is also useful in experimental settings.
- Ultrasonography allows for noninvasive abdominal assessment and enhances animal welfare via the reduction of painful diagnostic procedures.
- Reticular motility is used to exemplify how the forestomach function in calves progresses and gradually approaches that of adult cattle.

INTRODUCTION

Ultrasonographic findings of the reticulum, rumen, omasum, and abomasum of mature cattle were recently summarized and published.[1] The gastrointestinal tract of the calf undergoes significant changes associated with the development of the rumen and the transition from a milk-based to a roughage-based diet and differs from the tract of mature cattle. For this reason, ultrasonographic findings in mature cattle are not directly applicable to calves. In addition to ultrasonography, CT is useful for the assessment of the position, appearance, and size of intra-abdominal organs and their changes during development of the calf.[2–4] The aim of this review is to describe the abdominal organs in calves from birth to the age of 100 days. Calves used in ultrasonographic studies for the description of abdominal organs ranged in age from 0 to 14 days,[5] 16 to 33 days,[6,7] and 87 to 90 days.[6,8] To optimize the

The author has nothing to disclose.
Department of Farm Animals, University of Zurich, Winterthurerstrasse 260, Zurich CH-8057, Switzerland
E-mail address: ubraun@vetclinics.uzh.ch

Vet Clin Food Anim 32 (2016) 85–107
http://dx.doi.org/10.1016/j.cvfa.2015.09.011
0749-0720/16/$ – see front matter © 2016 Elsevier Inc. All rights reserved.

vetfood.theclinics.com

investigation of organ development in calves, a cohort of calves underwent serial ultrasonographic examination from birth to the age of 100 days.[9–11] The goal of that study was to monitor and describe the development of the reticulum, rumen, omasum, abomasum, spleen, liver, gall bladder, caudal vena cava, and portal vein in 6 healthy calves from birth to the age of 104 days.

TECHNIQUE OF ULTRASONOGRAPHIC EXAMINATION OF CALVES

A 5.0-MHz to 7.5-MHz linear or convex transducer is ideal,[7,11] but a transducer with a higher resolution, for instance 13.0 MHz, may be used for the examination of organ walls. The investigation of the motility of the forestomachs and abomasum during the ingestion of milk is facilitated by video recording using a recorder connected to the ultrasound machine. This allows for the continuous recording of all images and in-depth analysis at a later date. The examinations are conducted in the standing nonsedated animal. To improve contact between transducer and skin, the hair is clipped, the skin cleaned with alcohol, and obstetric lubricant is applied to the skin. A contact gel is also applied to the transducer.

RETICULUM
Examination of the Reticulum

The reticulum is examined in the ventral median and left and right ventral thoracic regions with the transducer held parallel to the longitudinal axis of the calf, and the reticulum is identified.[7,11] The contour and shape of the reticulum are assessed first and then the motility is recorded for 3 minutes. The number and the amplitude of contractions are recorded.

Ultrasonographic Findings of the Reticulum

The reticulum is rarely visualized in the first 2 weeks because it is very small and not close enough to the ventral abdominal wall to be within reach of the ultrasound beams.[5,9,11] From the third week, the reticulum can always be visualized in the sternal region. The spleen or the liver is often seen between the ventral abdominal wall and the reticulum until the age of approximately 80 days (**Fig. 1**). After the age of 100 days, the

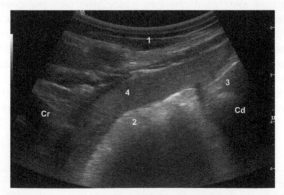

Fig. 1. Ultrasonogram of the reticulum in a 44-day-old Holstein Friesian calf imaged from the left paramedial sternal region using a 5-MHz convex transducer. 1, Ventral abdominal wall; 2, reticulum; 3, abomasum; 4, spleen; Cd, caudal; Cr, cranial. (*From* Braun U, Krüger S, Hässig M. Ultrasonographic examination of the reticulum, rumen, omasum and abomasum during the first 100 days of life in calves. Res Vet Sci 2013;95(2):328; with permission.)

reticulum is always adjacent to the ventral abdominal wall. The reticular wall appears as an echoic line, as described in mature cattle.[12] Because of its gaseous nature, the reticular content is not usually visible or it may appear as hypoechoic, cloudy, ill-defined material near the reticular wall. Small projections indicating the mucosal folds and the reticular honeycomb pattern are only seen in exceptional cases. Reticular contractions are biphasic similar to those seen in adult cattle.[12] During rumination, contractions are triphasic, as seen in adult cattle. The contraction preceding the normal biphasic contraction serves to transport the cud into the esophagus, from where it is propelled to the mouth and chewed. The frequency of reticular contractions increases significantly in the first 100 days of life; there were 0.9, 1.0, 1.2, 1.4, and 1.4 contractions per minute at the ages of 20, 40, 60, 80, and 100 days, respectively.[9,11]

The reticulum cannot be visualized in preweaned calves during and 30 minutes after ingestion of milk because it is displaced craniodorsally by the expanding abomasum and becomes obscured by the lungs.[6,7] The content and shape as well as the motility of the reticulum do not change during suckling. Likewise, the ultrasonographic appearance of the reticulum does not change during and after eating hay and grass silage but the frequency of contractions and the interval between contractions change significantly.[6,8] During feeding, the mean number of 10 calves during a 9-minute measuring period was 18.5, which was a significant increase from 11.1 before feeding and 11.5 after feeding. Because of the increased rate of contractions, the interval between contractions was significantly shorter ($P<.01$) during eating (21.7 seconds) than before (41.1 seconds) and after eating (37.3 seconds). The reticular contraction rate of 1.2 ± 0.23 contractions per minute in calves before feeding was similar to the rate in resting cows of 1.2 ± 0.13 contractions per minute[12] but slightly higher than the rate of 0.9 ± 0.19 contractions per minute in preweaned calves.[6,7] During feeding, the increase in the frequency of reticular contractions was greater in ruminating calves than in cows; in the former, it almost doubled from 1.2 to 2.1 contractions per minute and in the latter it increased from 1.2 to 1.6 contractions per minute.[12] The mean durations of the first and second contractions were 2.5 seconds and 3.9 seconds, respectively, in calves, which were similar to the values of 2.8 and 4.2 seconds measured in resting cows[12] and 2.4 and 4.9 seconds in preweaned calves.[6,7] Ruminating calves, preweaned calves, and cows differed with respect to the speed of the first reticular contraction; it was 7.0 cm/s in cows,[8] 3.5 cm/s in ruminating calves, and 1.7 cm/s in preweaned calves.[6,7] The approximately 4-fold increase from preweaned to ruminating calves to mature cows is an impressive illustration of the gradual reticular development in growing cattle.

RUMEN
Examination of the Rumen

The rumen is examined at the 6th to 12th intercostal spaces (ICSs) and the flank on both sides.[11] Each ICS and the flank are scanned from dorsal to ventral with the transducer held parallel to the ribs. The size of the rumen is determined by defining the dorsal and ventral visible margins of the rumen by measuring the distance from each margin to the dorsal midline using a tape measure. The size is then calculated by subtracting the distance of the dorsal margin from the distance of the ventral margin. The location of the longitudinal groove is identified to determine the size of the rumen sacs. The dorsal rumen sac extends from the dorsal visible margin to the longitudinal groove, and the ventral sac extends from the longitudinal sac to the ventral visible margin of the rumen. The thickness of the ruminal wall is best measured using a 13-MHz transducer.

Ultrasonographic Findings of the Rumen

The rumen can be visualized from the first day of life.[11] It is adjacent to the abdominal wall in the caudal abdomen and further cranially the spleen is seen between the abdominal wall and the rumen. The wall of the rumen is visible as an echoic line, and 3 layers, including the serosal, muscular, and mucosal tunics, can be clearly differentiated using the 13-MHz transducer. On the first day of life, the rumen content is anechoic with hyperechoic stippling and a small dorsal gas cap almost always can be seen. After the first day, most calves have reverberation artifacts dorsally (**Fig. 2**), indicating a gas cap, and an ingesta phase ventrally. The transition between the 2 phases is characterized by the abrupt disappearance of the reverberation artifact. Because of their gaseous nature, the ingesta and the ventral fluid phase cannot be seen. The ultrasonographic appearance of the rumen does not change in preweaned calves during and after the ingestion of milk[7] and in ruminating calves during and after eating hay and grass silage.[8]

The rumen is visible only from the left side on day 1 but from both sides thereafter. The longitudinal groove appears on the left as a mucosal fold, separating the dorsal and ventral sacs of the rumen, but the actual groove develops later (**Fig. 3**). Because of superimposition of the lung and spleen, the distance between the dorsal visible

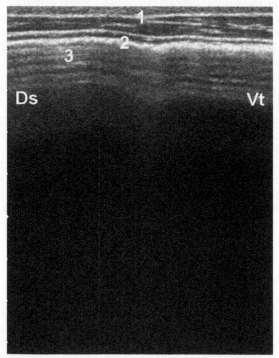

Fig. 2. Ultrasonogram of the dorsal sac of the rumen in a 3-month-old Brown Swiss calf viewed from the 11th ICS on the left side in the region of the dorsal gas cap using a 5.0-MHz linear transducer. 1, Lateral abdominal wall; 2, rumen wall; 3, reverberation artifacts at the level of the dorsal gas cap in the rumen; Ds, dorsal; Vt, ventral. (*From* Braun U, Krüger S, Hässig M. Ultrasonographic examination of the reticulum, rumen, omasum and abomasum during the first 100 days of life in calves. Res Vet Sci 2013;95(2):328; with permission.)

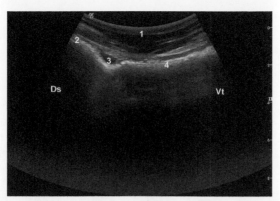

Fig. 3. Ultrasonogram of the rumen in a 44-day-old Holstein Friesian calf imaged from the 11th ICS on the left side using a 5-MHz convex transducer. 1, Lateral abdominal wall; 2, wall of the dorsal sac of rumen; 3, longitudinal groove; 4, wall of the ventral sac of rumen; Ds, dorsal; Vt, ventral. (*From* Braun U, Krüger S, Hässig M. Ultrasonographic examination of the reticulum, rumen, omasum and abomasum during the first 100 days of life in calves. Res Vet Sci 2013;95(2):328; with permission.)

margin of the rumen and the dorsal midline is largest in the 7th ICS (**Fig. 4**). It becomes smaller further caudally and is smallest in the 12th ICS. In the flank, the distance between the dorsal midline and the dorsal margin of the rumen increases. In contrast, the distance between the dorsal midline and the ventral visible margin of the rumen does not change much.

In each ICS, the overall size of the rumen increases progressively with age (**Fig. 5**). The most pronounced increase occurs after weaning, which was between days 60 and 80 in a study at the author's clinic. The same is true for the size of the dorsal and ventral sacs of the rumen. Until day 40, the dorsal and ventral sacs are similar in size, and after day 60, the ventral sac is slightly larger. The length of the rumen also increases gradually; on the first day, the rumen does not extend beyond the last rib but can be seen in the flank region from day 20. The cranial dorsal blind sac of the rumen cannot be seen

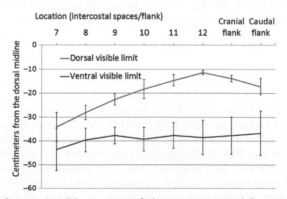

Fig. 4. Dorsal and ventral visible margins of the rumen imaged from the 7th ICS to the caudal flank on the left side in 6 62-day-old Holstein Friesian calves (examination 4; mean ± SD). (*From* Braun U, Krüger S, Hässig M. Ultrasonographic examination of the reticulum, rumen, omasum and abomasum during the first 100 days of life in calves. Res Vet Sci 2013;95(2):329; with permission.)

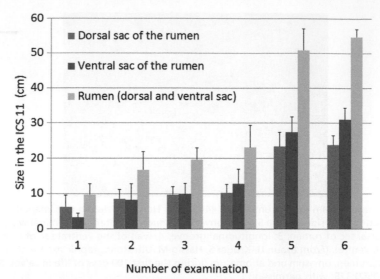

Fig. 5. Size of the dorsal and ventral ruminal sacs and the entire rumen imaged from the left side at the 11th ICS in 6 Holstein Friesian calves during the first 104 days of age (mean ± SD). Examination numbers 1, 2, 3, 4, 5, and 6 correspond to the ages of 2, 20, 41, 62, 83, and 99 days, respectively. (*From* Braun U, Krüger S, Hässig M. Ultrasonographic examination of the reticulum, rumen, omasum and abomasum during the first 100 days of life in calves. Res Vet Sci 2013;95(2):329; with permission.)

in the newborn but it appears as a semicircular structure between the reticulum and the ventral sac of the rumen from day 20, similar to descriptions in adult cattle. It contracts immediately after the biphasic reticular contraction.

OMASUM
Examination of the Omasum

The omasum is examined on the right side from all ICSs from dorsal to ventral with the transducer held parallel to the ribs.[7,11] The dorsal and ventral visible margins and the size of the omasum are determined analogous to the method used for the rumen.

Ultrasonographic Findings of the Omasum

The omasum can always be seen from the right side.[11] It is medial to the liver dorsally and usually medial to the small intestines ventrally and only occasionally directly adjacent to the abdominal wall. In the first few days of life, the omasum can occasionally also be seen from the 7th to 10th ICSs on the left side. It is seen on the right side from the 6th to 9th ICSs and occasionally from the 10th ICS. The best images are obtained at the 8th or 9th ICSs. In the newborn calf, the omasal wall usually appears as a completely circular line (**Fig. 6**). The omasal contents are echoic in these cases and the omasal leaves are seen as fine echoic lines. After a few days, the omasal contents can no longer be seen because of their gaseous nature, as described in adult cattle. The omasal wall then appears as a semicircular to circular echoic line (**Fig. 7**). Sometimes the origin of the omasal leaves can be seen as echoic projections protruding into the omasal lumen. The ultrasonographic appearance of the omasum remains unchanged in suckling calves during the ingestion of milk[7] and also in ruminating calves when they eat hay and grass silage.[8]

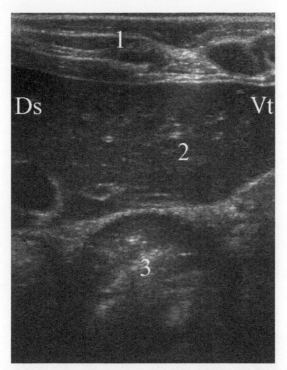

Fig. 6. Ultrasonogram of the omasum imaged from the 8th ICS in a 1-day-old Holstein Friesian calf. The omasum is circular and the omasal leaves are visible as distinct echoic lines. 1, Lateral abdominal wall; 2, liver; 3, omasum; Ds, dorsal; Vt, ventral. (*From* Krüger SS. Sonographische Untersuchungen an Haube, Pansen, Psalter, Labmagen, Milz und Leber von Kälbern von der Geburt bis zum Alter von 100 Tagen [dissertation]. Zurich (Switzerland): University of Zurich; 2012; with permission.)

The dorsal visible border of the omasum has a caudodorsal course (**Fig. 8**). It is furthest from the dorsal midline at the 6th ICS and moves progressively closer to the dorsal midline toward the 10th ICS. The visible omasal size measured at the 8th and 9th ICSs increases in the first 100 days, whereas the size measured in the 6th and 7th ICSs does not change appreciably (**Fig. 9**). The visible omasal size is largest in the 8th ICS and smallest in the 6th ICS. Typically, omasal motility cannot be detected.

ABOMASUM
Examination of the Abomasum

The abomasum is scanned from the 5th to the 12th ICSs and the flank on both sides starting at the ventral midline and progressing laterally and dorsally with the transducer held parallel to the ribs.[7,11] The location and size of the abomasum and visibility of its wall, folds, and content are assessed before and after the ingestion of milk. The abomasal length is measured in the ventral midline. Video recordings can be made of the abomasum slightly to the left of the ventral midline during and after the ingestion of milk to document filling of the abomasum and clotting of the milk. The time between the start of milk intake and the appearance of the milk in the abomasum can be measured using a stopwatch.

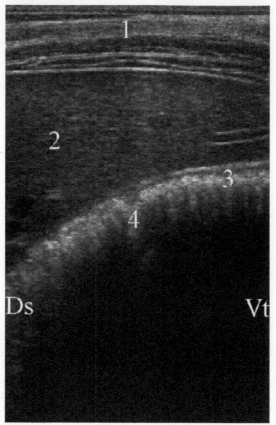

Fig. 7. Ultrasonogram of the omasum imaged from the 7th ICS in a 104-day-old Holstein Friesian calf. The omasum is medial to the liver and its wall is seen as an echoic convex line. The omasal leaves and the omasal content are not visible because of the gaseous nature of the latter. 1, Lateral abdominal wall; 2, Liver; 3, Omasum; 4, Insertion of an omasal leave; Ds Dorsal; Vt Ventral. (*From* Krüger SS. Sonographische Untersuchungen an Haube, Pansen, Psalter, Labmagen, Milz und Leber von Kälbern von der Geburt bis zum Alter von 100 Tagen [dissertation]. Zurich (Switzerland): University of Zurich; 2012; with permission.)

Ultrasonographic Findings of the Abomasum

The ultrasonographic appearance of the abomasum strongly depends on the time of milk intake. In the newborn calf, the abomasum is the largest organ and dominates the abdominal cavity. It is visible at the 5th to 12th ICSs and from the ventral flank. The content is heterogeneous and hypoechoic with hyperechoic stippling (**Fig. 10**) and often contains hyperechoic particles of varying size reflecting clotted milk. The abomasal wall appears as a fine echoic line and the abomasal folds are often distinct. From day 80 onward, the pyloric part of the abomasum can often be seen on the right side parallel to the fundic part of the stomach. The pylorus usually is oval to circular in cross section and has a characteristic spoke wheel appearance.[5]

The influx of milk is readily seen and first appears as a cloudlike hyperechoic mass. This expands to fill the entire abomasal lumen and is seen as homogeneous hyperechoic content (**Fig. 11**). In contrast to cow's milk, milk replacer appears heterogeneous and hyperechoic.[13] The mean interval between the start of nursing and the

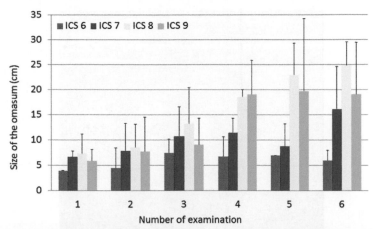

Fig. 8. Dorsal and ventral visible margins of the omasum imaged from the right side at the 6th to the 9th ICSs in 6 40-day-old Holstein Friesian calves (mean ± SD). For key for the examination numbers, see **Fig. 5**. (*From* Braun U, Krüger S, Hässig M. Ultrasonographic examination of the reticulum, rumen, omasum and abomasum during the first 100 days of life in calves. Res Vet Sci 2013;95(2):330; with permission.)

ultrasonographic appearance of milk in the abomasum varies from 10 to 25 seconds (range of individual examinations 5.9–68.0 seconds). After the influx of milk, the abomasal content usually appears as homogeneous, and rarely heterogeneous, hyperechoic material, and the abomasal folds are seen as distinct, undulating, echoic folds. Toward the end of nursing, the first signs of milk clotting can usually be seen in

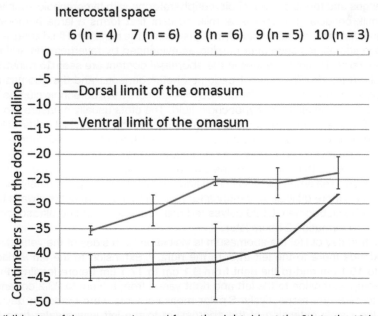

Fig. 9. Visible size of the omasum imaged from the right side at the 6th to the 10th ICSs in 6 Holstein Friesian calves from birth to 104 days of age (mean ± SD). (*From* Braun U, Krüger S, Hässig M. Ultrasonographic examination of the reticulum, rumen, omasum and abomasum during the first 100 days of life in calves. Res Vet Sci 2013;95(2):330; with permission.)

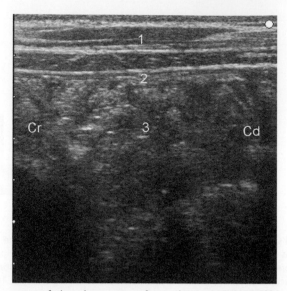

Fig. 10. Ultrasonogram of the abomasum of a Holstein Friesian calf before suckling. A 5.0-MHz linear transducer was used to scan the ventral abdomen. The ingesta appear heterogeneous and have echoic and hypoechoic components. 1, Ventral abdominal wall; 2, abomasal wall; 3, abomasal contents; Cd, caudal; Cr, cranial. (*From* Braun U, Gautschi A. Ultrasonography of the reticulum, rumen, omasum and abomasum in 10 calves before, during and after ingestion of milk. Schweiz Arch Tierheilkd 2012;154(7):293; with permission.)

the form of consolidation of the hyperechoic material. The homogeneous echoic content changes and forms a hypoechoic peripheral zone with hyperechoic stippling and echoic milk coagula. The abomasal milk content first forms a large homogeneous clump and distinct moving echoic stippling is seen in the peripheral fluid zone. A dorsal gas cap is sometimes seen after nursing as evidenced by reverberation artifacts on ultrasonograms. Distinct changes in the abomasal content are seen 15 minutes after milk intake (**Fig. 12**). The content becomes heterogeneous and the abomasal folds usually no longer can be seen. The clotted milk appears as hyperechoic clumps[6,7,14,15] surrounded by a small rim of hypoechoic fluid. The clots usually measure more than 5 cm in diameter. Thirty minutes after milk intake, the abomasal folds are again distinct. The visible clots are still the same size but they start to disintegrate and to become less distinct and overall less echoic, and the peripheral fluid rim becomes larger. By 2 hours after milk intake, the clumps are much smaller and their size varies from 1 to 5 cm. The amounts of solid and liquid contents are approximately the same. The pylorus is more difficult to identify after feeding than before but is always located in the right hemiabdomen. Of 29 calves fed milk replacer, 8 had no ultrasonographic signs of curd formation 2 hours later.[16]

On the first day of life, the abomasum is visible on both sides of the ventral midline but it extends more to the left than to the right.[11] Extension to the left varied from 8.9 cm to 15.1 cm and to the right from 3.1 cm to 17.1 cm before feeding (**Fig. 13**). After feeding, extension to the left and right varied from 8.9 cm to 23.2 cm and from 3.4 cm to 19.8 cm, respectively. Similar measurements were made on days 20 to 60 and the visible extension of the abomasum to the left was greater than that to the right (**Fig. 14**). From day 80 (the calves were weaned at day 60), abomasal extension to the left was smaller because of the expanding rumen. The visible extension to the right changed little in the first 100 days.

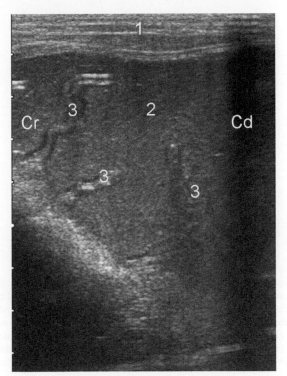

Fig. 11. Ultrasonogram of the abomasum of a Holstein Friesian calf during suckling. A 5.0-MHz linear transducer was used to scan the ventral abdomen. The ingested milk has not clotted yet and appears as a homogeneous mass. The abomasal folds are clearly visible. 1, Ventral abdominal wall; 2, milk that has just entered the abomasum; 3, abomasal folds; Cd, caudal; Cr, cranial. (*From* Braun U, Gautschi A. Ultrasonography of the reticulum, rumen, omasum and abomasum in 10 calves before, during and after ingestion of milk. Schweiz Arch Tierheilkd 2012;154(7):293; with permission.)

The mean visible abomasal length varied from 12.9 cm to 23.8 cm before feeding (**Fig. 15**) and changed little in the first 60 days. On day 100, the abomasal length was significantly greater ($P<.05$) than on day 1. With the exception of day 20, the visible abomasal length was greater before feeding than after feeding ($P<.05$).

Ultrasonographic measurements of abomasal dimensions (width, length, and height), location, and emptying rate were made in suckling calves before and after they were fed different volumes of milk replacer or oral electrolyte solutions.[14] All 3 abomasal dimensions increased during feeding, and after suckling, the abomasum was symmetrically located about the ventral midline. There were strong linear relationships between ultrasonographic and ingested volumes.

In contrast to feeding milk, the ultrasonographic appearance of the abomasum was the same before, during, and after feeding hay and grass silage.[8]

Ultrasonography was used to examine the effect of erythromycin, neostigmine, and metoclopramide on abomasal motility and emptying rate in suckling calves.[17] Six Holstein calves were examined 1 hour before until 3 hours after being fed milk replacer (60 mL/kg). The calves received 6 treatments of varying doses of the 3 drugs given 30 minutes before feeding. A high dose of erythromycin (8.8 mg/kg) increased the frequency of abomasal luminal pressure waves and the mean abomasal luminal pressure and decreased the half-time of abomasal emptying by 37%.

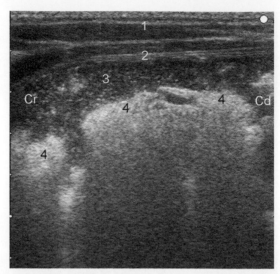

Fig. 12. Ultrasonogram of the abomasum of a Holstein Friesian calf 30 minutes after suckling, viewed from ventral using a 5.0-MHz linear transducer. The abomasal contents are heterogeneous and the clotted milk is seen as echoic clumps. Hypoechoic fluid is visible at the periphery of the abomasal lumen. 1, Ventral abdominal wall; 2, abomasal wall; 3, rim of hypoechoic fluid; 4, clotted milk; Cd, caudal; Cr, cranial. (*From* Braun U, Gautschi A. Ultrasonography of the reticulum, rumen, omasum and abomasum in 10 calves before, during and after ingestion of milk. Schweiz Arch Tierheilkd 2012;154(7):293; with permission.)

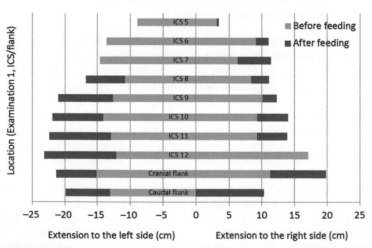

Fig. 13. Laterolateral extension of the abomasum before and after ingestion of milk imaged from the ventral abdominal wall from the 5th ICS to the flank (means) in 6 newborn Holstein Friesian calves. (*From* Braun U, Krüger S, Hässig M. Ultrasonographic examination of the reticulum, rumen, omasum and abomasum during the first 100 days of life in calves. Res Vet Sci 2013;95(2):331; with permission.)

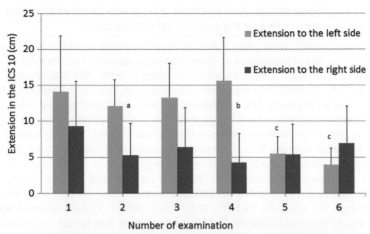

Fig. 14. Laterolateral extension of the abomasum before and after suckling imaged from the ventral abdominal wall at the level of the 10th ICS in 6 Holstein Friesian calves during the first 104 days of age (mean ± SD). [a,b] Difference between left and right ($P<.05$ and $<.01$, respectively). [c] Differences between examinations 4/5 and 4/6 ($P<.05$). For key for the examination numbers, see **Fig. 5**. (*From* Braun U, Krüger S, Hässig M. Ultrasonographic examination of the reticulum, rumen, omasum and abomasum during the first 100 days of life in calves. Res Vet Sci 2013;95(2):331; with permission.)

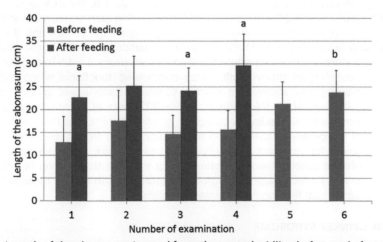

Fig. 15. Length of the abomasum imaged from the ventral midline before and after suckling in 6 Holstein Friesian calves during the first 104 days of age (mean ± SD). There are no post-suckling measurements at examinations 5 and 6 because the calves had been weaned. [a] Difference between before and after feeding ($P<.05$; paired t test). [b] Difference between examinations 1 and 6 ($P<.05$; paired t test). For key for the examination numbers, see **Fig. 5**. (*From* Braun U, Krüger S, Hässig M. Ultrasonographic examination of the reticulum, rumen, omasum and abomasum during the first 100 days of life in calves. Res Vet Sci 2013;95(2):331; with permission.)

ESOPHAGEAL GROOVE REFLEX AND FACTORS AFFECTING GROOVE CLOSURE
Ultrasonographic Monitoring of the Esophageal Groove Reflex

The term, *esophageal groove reflex*, refers to the reflex spiral contraction of 2 muscular folds forming the lips of the groove and simultaneous relaxation of the reticulo-omasal orifice and the omasal canal creating a bypass from the esophagus to the abomasum.[18] As a result, the ingested milk bypasses the reticulorumen and flows directly into the abomasum. The functioning of the esophageal groove reflex is easily monitored during suckling using ultrasonography; a functional reflex is confirmed when milk is seen entering the abomasum during milk intake.[7,14,19] Complete or partial failure of the reflex can result from unnatural housing and feeding management[18] or from neonatal disorders, such as diarrhea. Milk given to a calf by tube feeding is deposited into the reticulorumen.[20,21] When a healthy calf nurses, approximately 10% of the ingested milk reaches the reticulorumen[22] from where it is actively transported through the omasum into the abomasum within 3 hours without adversely affecting the forestomach system.[23] Milk remaining in the rumen for an extended period of time undergoes bacterial lactose fermentation leading to a disorder referred to as *ruminal drinker syndrome*.[24] Fermenting milk in the rumen of these calves can be detected ultrasonographically.[6,25]

Examination of the Esophageal Groove Reflex

Conditions required for a functional esophageal groove reflex include a normal health status, spontaneous suckling, normal odor and taste of the milk, and contact of the milk with relevant chemoreceptors in the oral cavity and esophagus.[24] Visual, auditory, and olfactory stimuli are also believed to be involved in esophageal groove closure.[26] The effect of the feeding method and other factors on esophageal groove closure were recently investigated in healthy calves.[13,19] The reflex was examined in milk-fed calves in the first 17 weeks of life. Other experiments were conducted to test the effect of various milk temperatures (20°C, 30°C, 39°C, and 45°C), different milk replacer concentrations (100, 125, and 150 g/L water), different feeding techniques (bucket feeding and different nipple positions), and different nipple openings (1 mm and 8 mm) on esophageal groove closure. The reticulum and abomasum were monitored ultrasonographically before, during, and after ingestion of milk using a 5-MHz convex transducer. The esophageal groove reflex was considered functional when milk was observed entering the abomasum during suckling. Esophageal groove closure occurred in all calves at each feeding in the first 17 weeks of life and in all calves at all examinations with all feeding techniques, at all milk temperatures, and with all milk replacer concentrations. It should not be concluded from these findings that feeding technique has no effect on esophageal groove closure. More likely, occasional deviation from the optimal feeding technique, for instance the feeding of cold milk, does not adversely affect esophageal groove closure but can lead to digestive disorders if the suboptimal feeding management persists.

RUMINAL DRINKER SYNDROME

Ultrasonographic examination of the reticulum is well suited for the differentiation of healthy calves and calves with ruminal drinker syndrome and to visualize the milk in the reticulorumen of the latter. In ruminal drinkers, the reticular wall appears as an echoic line,[25] as described in healthy calves,[7] but the 2 groups of calves differ with respect to the reticular content. Reticular content is not seen in healthy suckling calves[7] but appears as hyperechoic and heterogeneous material in ruminal drinkers (**Fig. 16**). Reticular folds are distinct in ruminal drinkers[25] and the honeycomb structure

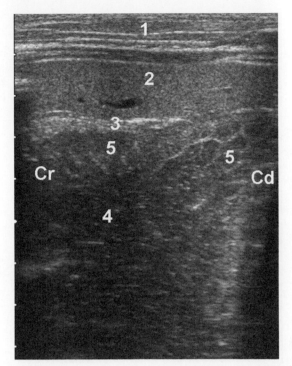

Fig. 16. Ultrasonogram of the reticulum of a 37-day-old Swiss Braunvieh calf with ruminal drinking syndrome. The 5.0-MHz linear transducer was held parallel to the sternum in the left lower thoracic area. The reticular content appears heterogeneous and echoic and the honeycomb-like structure of the mucosa can be seen. 1, Abdominal wall; 2, spleen; 3, reticular wall; 4, reticular content; 5, honeycomb-like structure of the mucosa, Cd, caudal; Cr, cranial. (*From* Braun U, Gautschi A. Ultrasonographic examination of the forestomachs and the abomasum in ruminal drinker calves. Acta Vet Scand 2013;55:1; with permission.)

of the mucosa is often clearly visible (**Fig. 17**). Reticular contractions are biphasic, as seen in healthy calves, and the parameters of reticular contractions are similar[25] to those seen in healthy suckling calves.[7] Reticular motility does not seem affected by the acidic and liquid content, although generally acidic rumen content has an adverse effect on forestomach motility in calves.[27,28]

Ultrasonography is useful for the detection of milk in the ventral sac of the rumen in ruminal drinkers. The level of milky fluid may reach the longitudinal groove or in exceptional cases into the dorsal sac of the rumen, and the fluid is hypoechoic and heterogeneous. The ruminal wall measures on average 3.5 mm near the longitudinal groove and 3.2 mm in the ventral sac compared with 2.2 and 1.7 mm, respectively, in healthy calves.[6,7,25] Ruminal drinkers and healthy calves do not differ in wall thickness of the dorsal sac of the rumen. The thickening of the ruminal wall in the lower ruminal region is a sequel of hyperkeratosis/parakeratosis and rumenitis, caused by increased butyric and lactic acid concentrations and characterized by epithelial loss, erosions, and necrosis of the ruminal mucosa.[24]

Of 10 calves with ruminal drinker syndrome, the ultrasonographic appearance of the rumen only changed in 5 during ingestion of milk[25]; the milk entering the rumen was seen as hyperechoic fluid mixing with the fluid already present.

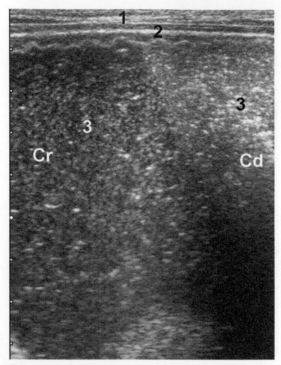

Fig. 17. Ultrasonogram of the ventral sac of the rumen of a 27-day-old Swiss Braunvieh calf with ruminal drinking syndrome. The 5.0-MHz linear transducer was held parallel to the ventral midline in the left lower abdominal area. The ruminal content appears heterogeneous and echoic. The undulating line medial to the ruminal wall indicates hyperkeratosis. 1, Ventral abdominal wall; 2, ruminal wall; 3, ruminal content; Cd, caudal; Cr, cranial. (*From* Braun U, Gautschi A. Ultrasonographic examination of the forestomachs and the aboasum in ruminal drinker calves. Acta Vet Scand 2013;55:1; with permission.)

The ultrasonographic findings of the omasum and abomasum were similar in ruminal drinkers and healthy suckling calves.[6,7,25] The omasal leaves were seen only occasionally in ruminal drinkers and the presence of a small amount of echoic fluid was the exception. The milk was seen entering the abomasum during suckling in all calves with ruminal drinker syndrome. As described for healthy suckling calves,[5,14,15] the abomasal content of ruminal drinkers undergoes successive changes associated with coagulation of the milk.

LIVER

Ultrasonography of the liver is of importance particularly in connection with a diagnosis of umbilical disorders.[29–32] For instance, the enlarged umbilical vein can be followed into the liver in calves with omphalophlebitis, and liver abscesses are readily detected.[29,31,32] Portosystemic shunt is rare in cattle but the shunt between the cranial mesenteric vein and the caudal vena cava could be directly visualized in an affected calf.[33]

Ultrasonographic Examination of the Liver

The liver of calves is scanned on the right side from the 5th ICS to the cranial flank from dorsal to ventral with the transducer held parallel to the ribs,[9,10] as described for adult cattle,[34] sheep,[35] and goats.[36] The liver parenchyma is first assessed subjectively by determining its echogenicity and the parenchymal pattern and whether the hepatic blood vessels can be visualized, and the appearance of the liver surface is assessed. The dorsal and ventral liver margins are identified in each ICS and the size of the liver is calculated, as described for adult cattle.[34] The thickness of the liver is measured in each ICS at the level of the portal vein using the electronic cursors on frozen images. The shape, position, and diameter of the caudal vena cava and portal vein and the shape, size, content, and appearance of the wall of the gallbladder are determined.

Ultrasonographic Findings of the Liver and Gallbladder

The parenchymal pattern of the liver consists of numerous fine echoes homogeneously distributed over the entire area of the organ (**Fig. 18**).[9,10] Branches of the portal vein and the hepatic veins in the parenchyma increase in size toward the portal vein and caudal vena cava, respectively. The wall of the portal vein is generally better defined than that of the hepatic veins because of an echoic rim, but clear differentiation is only possible in the area where stellar ramifications of the portal vein branch into the parenchyma. The intrahepatic bile ducts usually cannot be seen. The liver is always seen at the 5th to 12th ICSs and behind the last rib in healthy calves. Cranially it is adjacent to

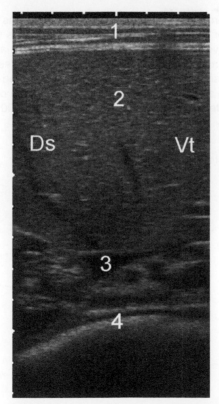

Fig. 18. Ultrasonogram of the liver and caudal vena cava viewed from the 11th ICS on the right side in a 95-day-old Holstein Friesian calf. 1, Abdominal wall; 2, liver; 3 caudal vena cava; 4, rumen; Ds, dorsal; Vt, ventral. (*From* Braun U, Krüger S. Ultrasonography of the spleen, liver, gallbladder, caudal vena cava and portal vein in healthy calves from birth to 104 days of age. Acta Vet Scand 2013;55:68; with permission.)

the diaphragm and dorsally there is superimposition of the lungs as far back as the 11th or 12th ICS. The dorsal visible margin of the liver runs parallel to the ventral border of the lungs from cranioventral to caudodorsal (**Fig. 19**). The distance of the dorsal visible margin of the liver from the dorsal midline decreases caudally because the liver becomes less obscured by the lung. The distance between the dorsal visible margin of the liver and the dorsal midline was greatest at the 5th ICS and shortest at the 11th ICS. The ventral visible margin had a similar course; it was furthest from the dorsal midline at the 5th ICS and closest to the dorsal midline at the cranial flank. The visible size of the liver is largest at the 8th to 11th ICSs and is considerably smaller cranially and caudally (**Fig. 20**). There is no measurable increase in liver size in the first 60 days, and the size is smaller at 80 days and 100 days than in the first 60 days. The thickness of the liver increases until day 40 and changes little thereafter until day 100 (**Fig. 21**). The maximum thickness is measured at the 8th and 9th ICSs.

The caudal vena cava is triangular in cross section, attributable to its location in the sulcus of the vena cava of the liver (see **Fig. 18**),[9,10] but occasionally is round to oval. The vein is always seen in at least one ICS, most commonly at the 9th to 12th ICSs, but is not seen cranial to these ICSs because of superimposition of the lungs. The mean circumference of the vein of newborn calves is largest at the 10th and 11th ICSs and varies from 3.8 cm to 4.3 cm. The circumference increases slightly and is largest at 6.5 cm at 40 days.

The portal vein is circular or oval in cross section and has stellate ramifications branching into the liver parenchyma (**Fig. 22**).[9,10] The wall is more echogenic than the wall of the caudal vena cava, and the portal vein is seen at more ICSs than the caudal vena cava because of a more ventral position and less superimposition of the lungs. It is always seen at the 7th to 11th ICSs. Compared with the caudal vena cava, the portal vein is always more ventral and closer to the diaphragmatic surface of the liver. The diameter of the vein varies little in the first 100 days (**Fig. 23**) and is

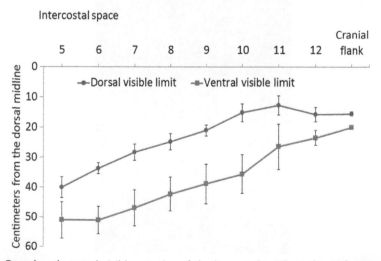

Fig. 19. Dorsal and ventral visible margins of the liver at the 5th to the 12th ICSs and the cranial flank on the right side in 6 Holstein Friesian calves (41.0 ± 0.76 days old; mean ± SD). (*From* Braun U, Krüger S. Ultrasonography of the spleen, liver, gallbladder, caudal vena cava and portal vein in healthy calves from birth to 104 days of age. Acta Vet Scand 2013;55:68; with permission.)

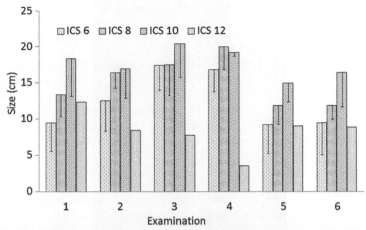

Fig. 20. Size of the liver (distance between the dorsal margin of the liver and the dorsal midline subtracted from the distance between the ventral margin of the liver and the dorsal midline) at the 6th to 12th ICSs in 6 healthy Holstein Friesian calves at examinations 1 to 6 (mean − SD). For key for the examination numbers, see **Fig. 5**. (*From* Braun U, Krüger S. Ultrasonography of the spleen, liver, gallbladder, caudal vena cava and portal vein in healthy calves from birth to 104 days of age. Acta Vet Scand 2013;55:68; with permission.)

smaller at the cranial ICSs than at the caudal ICSs. It ranges from 1.2 cm to 1.8 cm at the 9th to 11th ICSs.

The gallbladder is circular, oval, or pear-shaped (**Fig. 24**)[9,10] and sometimes extends beyond the ventral margin of the liver depending on the amount of bile. The content is anechoic and the wall is hyperechoic. The gallbladder can almost always be visualized, most commonly at the 9th ICS. It is often seen at more than one ICS and

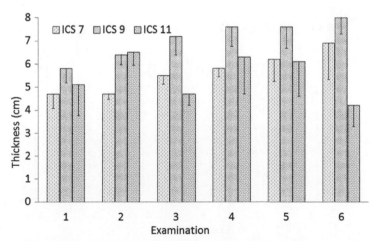

Fig. 21. Thickness of the liver at the 7th, 9th, and 11th ICSs in 6 healthy Holstein Friesian calves at examinations 1 to 6 (mean − SD). For key for the examination numbers, see **Fig. 5**. (*From* Braun U, Krüger S. Ultrasonography of the spleen, liver, gallbladder, caudal vena cava and portal vein in healthy calves from birth to 104 days of age. Acta Vet Scand 2013;55:68; with permission.)

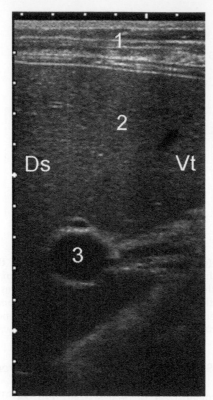

Fig. 22. Ultrasonogram of the portal vein viewed from the right side in an 83-day-old Holstein Friesian calf. 1, Abdominal wall; 2, liver parenchyma; 3, portal vein; Ds, dorsal, Vt, ventral. (*From* Braun U, Krüger S. Ultrasonography of the spleen, liver, gallbladder, caudal vena cava and portal vein in healthy calves from birth to 104 days of age. Acta Vet Scand 2013;55:68; with permission.)

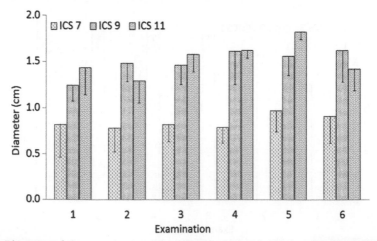

Fig. 23. Diameter of the portal vein at the 7th, 9th, and 11th ICSs in 6 healthy Holstein Friesian calves at examinations 1 to 6 (mean − SD). For key for the examination numbers, see **Fig. 5**. (*From* Braun U, Krüger S. Ultrasonography of the spleen, liver, gallbladder, caudal vena cava and portal vein in healthy calves from birth to 104 days of age. Acta Vet Scand 2013;55:68; with permission.)

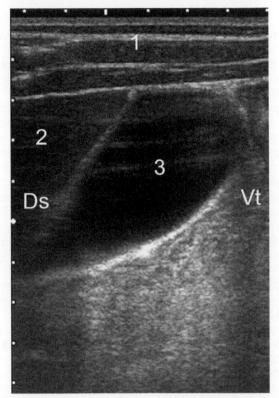

Fig. 24. Ultrasonogram of the gallbladder viewed from the right side in a 62-day-old Holstein Friesian calf. 1, Abdominal wall; 2, liver; 3, gallbladder; Ds, dorsal, Vt, ventral. (*From* Braun U, Krüger S. Ultrasonography of the spleen, liver, gallbladder, caudal vena cava and portal vein in healthy calves from birth to 104 days of age. Acta Vet Scand 2013;55:68; with permission.)

rarely at only 1 or at 3. The mean length varies from 1.5 cm to 5.5 cm and the mean width from 0.9 cm to 1.8 cm.

Abnormal Ultrasonographic Findings of the Liver and Gallbladder

Ultrasonographic changes of the liver in connection with umbilical disorders were recently described in detail.[32]

UMBILICUS

The ultrasonographic examination of the umbilicus and ultrasonographic findings in calves with umbilical disorders were recently described.[32]

SUMMARY

This article forms a guideline for the ultrasonographic examination of the abdomen in calves. Abdominal ultrasonography is primarily indicated for the assessment of the gastrointestinal tract of diseased calves but is also useful in experimental settings. Ultrasonography allows for noninvasive abdominal assessment and enhances animal welfare via the reduction of painful diagnostic procedures.

REFERENCES

1. Braun U. Ultrasonography of the gastrointestinal tract in cattle. Vet Clin North Am Food Anim Pract 2009;25(3):567–90.
2. Braun U, Schnetzler C, Ohlerth S, et al. Computed tomography of the abdomen of calves during the first 105 days of life: I. Reticulum, rumen, omasum and abomasum. Schweiz Arch Tierheilkd 2014;156(5):217–25.
3. Braun U, Schnetzler C, Augsburger H, et al. Computed tomography of the abdomen of calves during the first 105 days of life: II. liver, spleen, and small and large intestines. Schweiz Arch Tierheilkd 2014;156(5):227–36.
4. Braun U, Schnetzler C, Augsburger H, et al. Computed tomography of the abdomen of calves during the first 105 days of life: III. Urinary tract and adrenal glands. Schweiz Arch Tierheilkd 2014;156(5):237–47.
5. Jung C. Sonographie der Lunge und des Abdomens beim bovinen Neonaten unter besonderer Berücksichtigung pathologischer Veränderungen [dissertation]. Giessen (Germany): Justus-Liebig-University of Giessen; 2002.
6. Gautschi A. Sonographische Untersuchungen an Haube, Pansen, Psalter und Labmagen von 30 Kälbern [dissertation]. Zurich (Switzerland): University of Zurich; 2010.
7. Braun U, Gautschi A. Ultrasonography of the reticulum, rumen, omasum and abomasum in 10 calves before, during and after ingestion of milk. Schweiz Arch Tierheilkd 2012;154(7):287–97.
8. Braun U, Gautschi A, Tschuor A, et al. Ultrasonography of the reticulum, rumen, omasum and abomasum before, during and after ingestion of hay and grass silage in 10 calves. Res Vet Sci 2012;93(3):1407–12.
9. Krüger SS. Sonographische Untersuchungen an Haube, Pansen, Psalter, Labmagen, Milz und Leber von Kälbern von der Geburt bis zum Alter von 100 Tagen [dissertation]. Zurich (Switzerland): University of Zurich; 2012.
10. Braun U, Krüger S. Ultrasonography of the spleen, liver, gallbladder, caudal vena cava and portal vein in healthy calves from birth to 104 days of age. Acta Vet Scand 2013;55:68.
11. Braun U, Krüger S, Hässig M. Ultrasonographic examination of the reticulum, rumen, omasum and abomasum during the first 100 days of life in calves. Res Vet Sci 2013;95(2):326–33.
12. Braun U, Rauch S. Ultrasonographic evaluation of reticular motility during rest, eating, rumination and stress in 30 healthy cows. Vet Rec 2008;163(19):571–4.
13. Brammertz C. Überprüfung der Schlundrinnenfunktion bei Kälbern, Rinder und Kühen mittels sonographischer Untersuchung [dissertation]. Zurich (Switzerland): University of Zurich; 2014.
14. Wittek T, Constable PD, Marshall T, et al. Ultrasonographic measurement of abomasal volume, location, and emptying rate in calves. Am J Vet Res 2005; 66(3):537–44.
15. Miyazaki T, Miyazaki M, Yasuda J, et al. Ultrasonographic imaging of abomasal curd in preruminant calves. Vet J 2009;179(1):109–16.
16. Miyazaki T, Miyazaki M, Yasuda J, et al. No abomasal curd formation in preruminant calves after ingestion of a clotting milk replacer. Vet J 2010;183(2):205–9.
17. Wittek T, Constable PD. Assessment of the effects of erythromycin, neostigmine, and metoclopramide on abomasal motility and emptying rate in calves. Am J Vet Res 2005;66(3):545–52.
18. Kaske M. Motorik des Magen-Darm-Kanals. In: Engelhardt W, Breves G, editors. Physiologie der Haustiere. Stuttgart (Germany): Enke Verlag; 2010. p. 347–79.

19. Braun U, Brammertz C. Ultrasonographic examination of the oesophageal groove reflex in young calves under various feeding conditions. Schweiz Arch Tierheilkd 2015;157(8):457–63.
20. Schipper IA, Colville T, Samuel CW, et al. The effects of intubation feeding of the newborn calf. Farm Res 1984;42(2):14–7.
21. Dirksen G, Baur T. Pansenazidose beim Milchkalb infolge Zwangsfütterung. Tierärztl Umsch 1991;46(1):257–61.
22. Ruckebusch V, Kay RNB. Sur le réflexe de fermeture de la gouttière oesophagienne. Ann Biol Anim Biochim Biophys 1971;11(2):281.
23. Lateur-Rowet HJM, Breukink HJ. The failure of the oesophageal groove reflex, when fluids are given with an oesophageal feeder to newborn and young calves. Vet Q 1983;5(2):68–74.
24. Dirksen G. Krankheiten von Haube und Pansen bei Milchkalb und Jungrind. In: Dirksen G, Gründer HD, Stöber M, editors. Innere Medizin und Chirurgie des Rindes. Berlin: Parey Buchverlag; 2002. p. 455–69.
25. Braun U, Gautschi A. Ultrasonographic examination of the forestomachs and the abomasum in ruminal drinker calves. Acta Vet Scand 2013;55:1.
26. Abe M, Iriki T, Kondoh K, et al. Effects of nipple or bucket feeding of milk-substitute on rumen by-pass and on rate of passage in calves. Br J Nutr 1979; 41(1):175–81.
27. Breukink HJ, Wensing T, Van Weeren-Keverling Buisman A, et al. Consequences of failure of the reticular groove reflex in veal calves fed milk replacer. Vet Q 1988; 10(2):126–35.
28. Bättig U, Regi G, Stocker H. Pansensaft-Untersuchung bei Kälbern mit gestörter und normaler Sauglust. Tierärztl Prax 1992;22(1):44–8.
29. Lischer CJ, Steiner A. Ultrasonography of the umbilicus in calves. Part 2: ultrasonography, diagnosis and treatment of umbilical diseases. Schweiz Arch Tierheilkd 1994;136(6–7):227–41.
30. Heidemann A, Grunert E. Ultraschalldiagnostik als Entscheidungshilfe für das weitere Vorgehen bei Nabelentzündungen des neugeborenen Kalbes. Prakt Tierarzt 1995;76(9):742–6.
31. Flöck M. Ultraschalldiagnostik von Entzündungen der Nabelstrukturen, persistierendem Urachus und Umbilikalhernie beim Kalb. Berl Münch Tierärztl Wschr 2003;116(1–2):2–11.
32. Steiner A, Lejeune B. Ultrasonographic assessment of umbilical disorders. Vet Clin North Am Food Anim Pract 2009;25(3):781–93.
33. Buczinski S, Duval J, D'Anjou MA, et al. Portocaval shunt in a calf: clinical, pathologic, and ultrasonographic findings. Can Vet J 2007;48(4):407–10.
34. Braun U, Gerber D. Influence of age, breed, and stage of pregnancy on hepatic ultrasonographic findings in cows. Am J Vet Res 1994;55(9):1201–5.
35. Braun U, Hausammann K. Ultrasonographic examination of the liver in sheep. Am J Vet Res 1992;53(2):198–202.
36. Braun U, Steininger K. Ultrasonographic characterization of the liver, caudal vena cava, portal vein, and gallbladder in goats. Am J Vet Res 2011;72(2):219–25.

Ultrasonographic Examination of the Spinal Cord and Collection of Cerebrospinal Fluid from the Atlanto-Occipital Space in Cattle

Ueli Braun, Prof Dr Med Vet, Dr Med Vet H C*, Jeannette Attiger, Med Vet

KEYWORDS

- Cattle • Ultrasonography • Spinal cord • Atlanto-occipital space
- Cerebrospinal fluid

KEY POINTS

- The spinal cord and its surrounding structures can readily be identified using ultrasonography.
- It is possible to collect cerebrospinal fluid (CSF) without blood contamination.
- Ultrasound guidance eliminates the need for marked ventroflexion of the head, which in turn minimizes defensive reactions that commonly occur when the blind technique is used.
- Ultrasound-guided collection of CSF is convenient and safe, and therefore, the method of choice for collection of CSF in cattle.

INTRODUCTION

The examination of cerebrospinal fluid (CSF) plays a major role in the diagnosis of central nervous system diseases in cattle. There are 2 sites from which CSF can be collected in cattle: the first is the atlanto-occipital (AO) space and the second is the lumbosacral foramen (LSF).[1,2] The exact site of needle insertion at both locations is determined by skeletal landmarks, but puncture is carried out blindly without visualization of the subarachnoid space.[1-4] For collection from the AO space, the head is ventroflexed at a 90° angle and the needle is inserted at the intersection between the dorsal midline and an imaginary line connecting the cranial edges of the wings

The authors have nothing to disclose.
Department of Farm Animals, University of Zurich, Winterthurerstrasse 260, CH-8057 Zurich, Switzerland
* Corresponding author.
E-mail address: ubraun@vetclinics.uzh.ch

of the atlas[2,4] or slightly cranial to that intersection.[1] A spinal needle is introduced into the subarachnoid space parallel to the longitudinal axis of the flexed head.[1,4] The depth to which the needle is inserted is not exactly predictable, and the needle is advanced slowly and carefully and monitored for free flow of CSF by removing the stylet at regular intervals.[2] Puncture of the spinal cord must be avoided because it can lead to nerve damage or even death of the patient.[2,5] Strong ventroflexion of the head required for this technique often provokes avoidance movements in the animal and may impair respiration. Furthermore, blind aspiration of CSF from the AO space frequently results in contamination of the sample with blood,[6,7] which can impair the diagnosis.[8–12] Finally, the spinal cord may be punctured during blind aspiration despite the precautions outlined above and results in pain evidenced by violent twitching. Based on experiences in the collection of CSF under ultrasonographic guidance in the horse,[13–15] the spinal canal of cattle was examined ultrasonographically and the feasibility of ultrasound-guided collection of CSF was investigated.[16,17] Another study described the ultrasonographic findings of diplomyelia of the lumbar spine in a calf,[18] and the ultrasonographic examination of the spinal cord in healthy calves was presented.[19] The purpose of this article is to describe the ultrasonographic findings of the spinal cord and its surrounding structures and the ultrasound-guided collection of CSF from the AO space in cattle.

ANATOMY OF THE ATLANTO-OCCIPITAL SPACE

The AO space is bordered by the occiput cranially and by the atlas caudally and is covered by the skin, the nuchal ligament, various muscles, and the AO membrane.[2,20] Ventral to this membrane is the cranial-most section of the vertebral canal, which contains the spinal cord surrounded by 3 meninges. The outermost meninx is the dura mater, which is separated from the vertebral periosteum by the epidural space.[21] The middle meninx is the dura arachnoidea, which is enveloped by the dura mater and consists of 3 layers. The outermost layer is made up of fibrocytes and collagen fibers and is separated from the dura mater by a so-called neurothelium. Avascular bundles of collagen fibers covered by neurothelium, referred to as arachnoid trabeculae, connect the outer layer with the inner layer of the dura arachnoidea, which also consists of collagen fibers and fibrocytes.[21,22] These trabeculae are in the middle layer and form a spider web-like network surrounded by CSF. The middle layer of the dura arachnoidea is referred to as the subarachnoid space[22] and contains the arteries that supply the central nervous system.[21] The innermost layer of the dura arachnoidea follows the superficial surface of the brain and spinal cord, whereas the outermost layer, together with the dura mater, forms a straight sac, which envelops the spinal cord. The innermost meninx, the pia mater, adheres to the surface of the brain and spinal cord and closely follows their contours. CSF-filled spaces, referred to as subarachnoid cisternae, are formed in the regions where the dura arachnoidea and pia mater separate over depressions in the brain or spinal cord. The cerebellomedullary cistern, also called the cisterna magna, is formed between the caudal aspect of the cerebellum and the medulla oblongata and in most domestic animals is of clinical importance for the collection of CSF from the AO space.[21,22] However, in cattle, the cerebellomedullary cistern cannot be accessed because of the caudal elongation of the occipital bone, and therefore, the caudal extension of the cistern, is punctured for collection of CSF.[23] The pia mater consists of loose connective tissue including blood vessels and nerves. It is tightly associated with the surface of the brain and spinal cord and is adjacent to the superficial glial cells of the central nervous system. The pia mater forms 2 narrow fibrous strips on either side of the spinal cord, called denticulate ligaments, with extensions that attach to the dura mater and provide stability to the spinal cord within the dural sac.[21,22]

The spinal cord is a cylindrical structure characterized by a dorsal median sulcus, 2 dorsolateral sulci, and a deep ventral median fissure. The dorsal afferent nerve roots enter the spinal cord at the dorsolateral sulci, and the efferent nerve roots exit the spinal cord ventrolaterally on both sides. The dorsal and ventral nerve roots unite in the subarachnoid space to form the spinal nerves, which exit the spinal canal through the intervertebral foramina. In the center of the spinal cord is the central canal, which is continuous with the ventricular system of the brain.[22]

ULTRASONOGRAPHIC EXAMINATION OF THE SPINAL CORD FROM THE ATLANTO-OCCIPITAL SPACE

The ultrasonographic findings of the spinal cord and the collection of CSF under ultrasonographic guidance from the AO space in 73 cows immediately after euthanasia and in 14 live cattle of various ages with central nervous disease were described.[16,17]

Preparation of Cattle for the Ultrasonographic Examination

For ultrasonographic examination and collection of CSF, cattle are placed in lateral recumbency. Cows are sedated with 0.07 to 0.10 mg/kg xylazine intravenously, followed by 0.05 mg/kg xylazine intramuscularly depending on the level of sedation. The cow is then placed on a tilt table and all 4 legs and the head are secured with straps. A 15 cm × 10 cm area over the AO space is clipped and cleaned with ethanol. The head is fixed to the table with a halter in mild ventroflexion (about 30°) to improve the ultrasonographic visibility of the spinal cord. Rarely, moderate ventroflexion of about 45° is required for successful imaging of the spinal cord and CSF collection, but strong ventroflexion of 90°, which is needed for blind CSF aspiration, is never required.

Technique of Ultrasonographic Examination

A 5.0- to 7.5-MHz linear or convex transducer is used, and after the application of conductive gel, the spinal cord and its surrounding structures are imaged in longitudinal and cross-section.

Ultrasonographic Findings of the Atlanto-Occipital Space

Ultrasonograms of the AO space show, from dorsal to ventral, the skin, the nuchal ligament, various muscles including the rectus capitis minor und major muscles, the AO membrane, and the vertebral canal, which is bordered by the hyperechoic dura mater. In longitudinal section, the muscles appear as echoic structures with longitudinal striations, and the nuchal ligament is hypoechoic. The spinal cord is seen as a hypoechoic band, some areas of which have a heterogeneous internal structure (**Fig. 1**). It is surrounded dorsally (toward the skin) as well as ventrally (away from the skin) by the subarachnoid space and is anechoic to hypoechoic and sometimes has a heterogeneous internal structure. Blood vessels often seen dorsolateral and adjacent to the dural sac can be interpreted as a venous sinus based on findings in the horse.[13] In cross-section, the spinal cord is circular and surrounded by the subarachnoid space (**Fig. 2**). The hyperechoic denticulate ligaments are often seen on both sides of the spinal cord between the pia mater and dura mater. The central canal is frequently seen as a hyperechoic spot in the middle of the spinal cord. The pia mater appears as an echoic line adjacent to the spinal cord. The dura mater and arachnoid membrane are also seen as a hyperechoic line but cannot be differentiated.

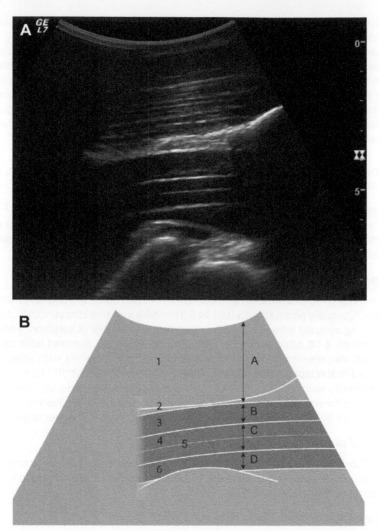

Fig. 1. Longitudinal ultrasonogram (*A*) and schematic representation (*B*) of the vertebral canal at the level of the AO space obtained immediately after euthanasia in a 3.5-year-old Swiss Braunvieh cow. Left is cranial and right is caudal. (1) Nuchal ligament, major and minor rectus capitis muscles; (2) AO membrane; (3) Subarachnoid space dorsal to the spinal cord; (4) Spinal cord; (5) Central canal; (6) Subarachnoid space ventral to the spinal cord; (A) Distance between skin and arachnoidea; (B) Depth of the subarachnoid space dorsal to the spinal cord; (C) Diameter of the spinal cord; (D) Depth of the subarachnoid space ventral to the spinal cord.

Measurements in the Atlanto-Occipital Space in 73 Euthanized Cows

The ultrasonographically visible structures were measured to generate reference intervals for the cows with central nervous system disorders.[16,17] Optimal sagittal and transverse ultrasonograms were frozen, and various variables were measured using the electronic cursors. The measurements made in the longitudinal and transverse planes are very similar (**Table 1**). In the longitudinal section, the distance between the skin and arachnoidea ranges from 30 to 52 mm (mean ± SD = 38.6 ± 4 mm), and the height of the subarachnoid spaces dorsal and ventral to the spinal cord

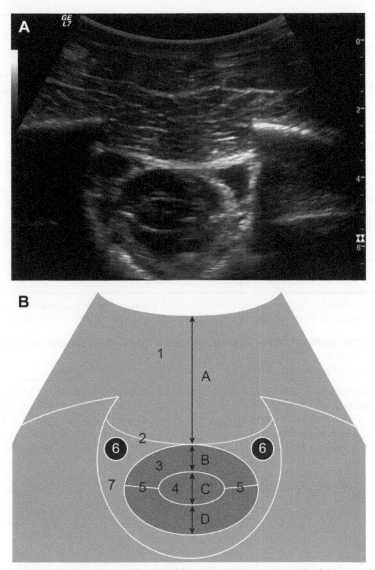

Fig. 2. Transverse ultrasonogram (*A*) and schematic representation (*B*) of the vertebral canal at the level of the AO space obtained immediately after euthanasia in a 3.5-year-old Swiss Braunvieh cow. (1) Nuchal ligament, major and minor rectus capitis muscles; (2) AO membrane; (3) Subarachnoid space; (4) Spinal cord; (5) Denticulate ligaments; (6) Venous sinus within the epidural space; (7) Epidural space; (A) Distance between skin and arachnoidea; (B) Depth of the subarachnoid space dorsal to the spinal cord; (C) Diameter of the spinal cord; (D) Depth of the subarachnoid space ventral to the spinal cord.

ranges from 5 to 12 mm (8.9 ± 1.6 mm) and from 4 to 11 mm (median = 8.4 mm), respectively. The height of the spinal cord varies from 6 to 13 mm (9.9 ± 1.2 mm) and the height of the entire dural sac varies from 20 to 34 mm (26.9 ± 3 mm). The spinal cord can be seen in the sagittal plane over a distance of 19 to 72 mm (43.1 ± 10.3 mm).

Table 1
Ultrasonographic measurements of the vertebral canal at the atlanto-occipital space in 73 euthanized cattle (mm, mean ± standard deviation, median, range)

Variable	Section	
	Longitudinal	Transverse
Distance between skin and arachnoidea	38.6 ± 4 (30–52) n = 68	39.5 ± 4.2 (32–52) n = 73
Depth of the subarachnoid space dorsal to the spinal cord	8.9 ± 1.6 (5–12) n = 67	9.2 ± 1.6 (6–13) n = 73
Diameter of spinal cord	9.9 ± 1.2 (6–13) n = 67	10.1 (8–15) n = 72
Depth of the subarachnoid space ventral to the spinal cord	8.4 (4–11) n = 68	8.8 ± 1.8 (5–14) n = 73
Diameter of entire dural sac	26.9 ± 3 (20–34) n = 68	28.2 ± 3.5 (21–40) n = 73
Length of visible spinal cord	43.1 ± 10.3 (19–72) n = 67	—

From Braun U, Attiger J, Brammertz C. Ultrasonographic examination of the spinal cord and collection of cerebrospinal fluid from the atlanto-occipital space in cattle. BMC Vet Res 2015;11:227.

ULTRASOUND-GUIDED COLLECTION OF CEREBROSPINAL FLUID FROM THE ATLANTO-OCCIPITAL SPACE
Preparation of Cattle and Cerebrospinal Fluid Collection Technique

After ultrasonography, the clipped area over the AO space is cleaned with iodine soap and disinfected, and the skin at the site of puncture is anesthetized using 5 mL of 2% lidocaine. The so-called freehand technique[24] with a spinal needle (0.90 × 90 mm, Terumo Spinal needle; Terumo Medical Corporation, Somerset, NJ, USA) is used to puncture the arachnoidea under ultrasonographic guidance (**Figs. 3** and **4**). Positioning

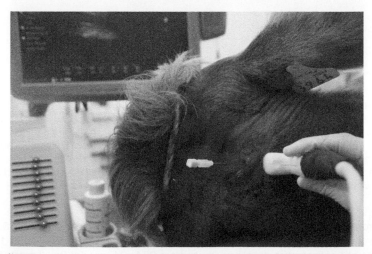

Fig. 3. Collection of CSF in a sedated cow in lateral recumbency. The head and legs are tied to the operating table. The fluid is collected from the AO space using a spinal needle and ultrasonographic guidance provided by a 5-MHz convex transducer.

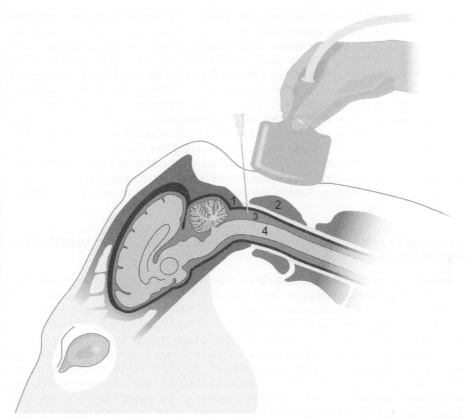

Fig. 4. Schematic diagram of puncture of the subarachnoid space for collection of CSF. The diagram is based on MRI images of the head of a 10-year-old Simmental cow. (1) Occiput; (2) Atlas; (3) Subarachnoid space; (4) Spinal cord.

the needle so that it is aligned perfectly with the sagittal orientation of the sound waves can pose a problem initially, but this technique becomes easier with practice, and the accidental puncture of blood vessels can be avoided. The needle is introduced in the median plane in a caudoventral direction. As described for CSF collection in the horse, the angle between the needle and the dura mater is critical.[13,15] When the angle is too small, the needle does not perforate the dura mater but pushes it ventrally. This complication has occurred regardless of the angle of the needle and is referred to as tenting in human medicine.[25] The tenting phenomenon increases the risk of accidental puncture of the spinal cord and must be avoided at all costs. After perforation of the arachnoidea and observation of the tip of the needle in the subarachnoid space, the stylet is removed and 3 to 5 mL of CSF is aspirated using a syringe. If the attempt is unsuccessful, the stylet is reinserted and the needle withdrawn partly or completely, and the puncture is repeated at a slightly different angle. A new needle is used after accidental puncture of a blood vessel or aspiration of blood. When done correctly and without spinal cord puncture, this technique does not elicit pain or avoidance behavior in cows.

Examination of the Cerebrospinal Fluid

Ultrasound-guided collection of CSF reduces the incidence of contamination of the CSF with blood, which is common when the blind puncture technique is used.[6,7]

Therefore, most CSF samples are clear and colorless, but it must be remembered that blood contamination is not always recognized macroscopically.[7,9,10] In CSF samples collected under ultrasound guidance at the authors' clinic, the red blood cell count ranged from 0 to 820 erythrocytes/µL CSF (median = 2.5 erythrocytes/µL CSF) **(Fig. 5)**. A minimum erythrocyte count of about 2000 to 3000 cells/µL is required to render a CSF sample grossly discolored or turbid,[8,9,26] which explains why practically all of the samples appeared uncontaminated. It also means that CSF collected using the described technique is well suited for diagnostic purposes in cattle with central nervous system disease. It should also be noted that it is possible to collect a clean CSF sample in a second attempt after a blood vessel has been punctured and hemorrhagic CSF is aspirated initially. This technique is a major advantage over the blind puncture technique, which usually does not allow for the collection of a blood-free CSF sample at the same collection site once a hemorrhagic sample or frank blood has been aspirated.

ULTRASONOGRAPHIC EXAMINATION OF THE SPINAL CORD FROM THE LUMBOSACRAL AREA IN THE CALF

In calves, the spinal cord also can be examined ultrasonographically between the 5th and 6th lumbar vertebrae or from the LSF,[18,19] but a detailed description of this technique in adult cows was not available at the time of this writing. There are anecdotal reports that lateral ultrasonograms of the spinal cord can be obtained at the LSF in adult cows. A 7.5-MHz linear transducer is best suited for the examination in calves. The calf is placed in lateral recumbency and positioned such that the lumbar vertebrae are slightly arched dorsally. Similar to the technique described for the AO space, the spinal cord and the surrounding structures are examined in the sagittal and transverse planes. The ultrasonographic appearance of the spinal cord is analogous to that at the AO space except that 2 spinal nerves are seen on transverse images. This technique allows for the diagnosis of spinal cord malformations, for instance, diplomyelia, which is the duplication of the spinal cord, including the central canal.[27]

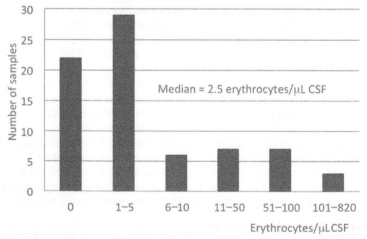

Fig. 5. Frequency distribution of different levels of blood contamination of CSF collected under ultrasound guidance in 73 cows.

SUMMARY

The spinal cord and its surrounding structures can readily be identified using ultrasonography. Also, it is possible to collect CSF without blood contamination. In addition, ultrasound guidance eliminates the need for marked ventroflexion of the head, which in turn minimizes defensive reactions that commonly occur when the blind technique is used. Ultrasound-guided collection of CSF is convenient and safe, and therefore, the method of choice for collection of CSF in cattle.

REFERENCES

1. Vandevelde M, Jaggy A, Lang J. Spezielle Untersuchungsmethoden. Untersuchung des Liquor Cerebrospinalis (LCS); Entnahmetechnik. In: Vandevelde M, Jaggy A, Lang J, editors. Veterinärmedizinische Neurologie. Ein Leitfaden für Studium und Praxis. Berlin: Parey Buchverlag; 2001. p. 63–9.
2. De Lahunta A, Glass E. Cerebrospinal fluid and hydrocephalus. In: De Lahunta A, Glass EN, editors. Veterinary neuroanatomy and clinical neurology. St Louis (MO): Saunders Elsevier; 2009. p. 54–76.
3. Di Terlizzi R, Platt SR. The function, composition and analysis of cerebrospinal fluid in companion animals: part II – analysis. Vet J 2009;180(1):15–32.
4. Kumar V, Kumar N. Diagnostic value of cerebrospinal fluid evaluation in veterinary practice: an overview. J Adv Vet Res 2012;2(3):213–7.
5. Luján Feliu-Pascual A, Garosi L, Dennis R, et al. Iatrogenic brainstem injury during cerebellomedullary cistern puncture. Vet Radiol Ultrasound 2008;49(5):467–71.
6. Averill DR. Examination of the cerebrospinal fluid. In: Kirk RW, editor. Current veterinary therapy: V. Small animal practice. Philadelphia: WB Saunders Company; 1974. p. 645–8.
7. Kornhuber ME, Kornhuber J, Kornhuber AW, et al. Positive correlation between contamination by blood and amino acid levels in cerebrospinal fluid of the rat. Neurosci Lett 1986;69(2):212–5.
8. Ylitalo P, Heikkinen ER, Myllylä VV. Evaluation of sucessive collections of cisternal cerebrospinal fluid in rats, rabbits, and cats. Exp Neurol 1976;50(2):330–6.
9. Miller MM, Sweeney CR, Russell GE, et al. Effects of blood contamination of cerebrospinal fluid on western blot analysis for detection of antibodies against Sarcocystis neurona and on albumin quotient and immunoglobulin G index in horses. J Am Vet Med Assoc 1999;215(1):67–71.
10. Sweeney CR, Russell GE. Differences in total protein concentration, nucleated cell count, and red blood cell count among sequential samples of cerebrospinal fluid from horses. J Am Vet Med Assoc 2000;217(1):54–7.
11. Finno CJ, Packham AE, Wilson WD, et al. Effects of blood contamination of cerebrospinal fluid on results of indirect fluorescent antibody tests for detection of antibodies against Sarcocystis neurona and Neospora hughesi. J Vet Diagn Invest 2007;19(3):286–9.
12. Doyle C, Solano-Gallego L. Cytologic interpretation of canine cerebrospinal fluid samples with low total nucleated cell concentration, with and without blood contamination. Vet Clin Pathol 2009;38(3):392–6.
13. Audigié F, Tapprest J, Didierlaurent D, et al. Ultrasound-guided atlanto-occipital puncture for myelography in the horse. Vet Radiol Ultrasound 2004;45(4):340–4.
14. Pease A, Behan A, Bohart G. Ultrasound-guided cervical centesis to obtain cerebrospinal fluid in the standing horse. Vet Radiol Ultrasound 2012;53(1):92–5.

15. Depecker M, Bizon-Mercier C, Couroucé-Malblanc A. Ultrasound-guided atlanto-occipital puncture for cerebrospinal-fluid analysis on the standing horse. Vet Rec 2014;174(2):45.
16. Attiger J. Liquorentnahme aus dem Spatium Atlanto-Occipitale unter Ultraschall-kontrolle beim Rind. Master-Thesis, University of Zurich; 2014.
17. Braun U, Attiger J, Brammertz C. Ultrasonographic examination of the spinal cord and collection of cerebrospinal fluid from the atlanto-occipital space in cattle. BMC Vet Res 2015;11:227.
18. Testoni S, Franz S, Dalla Pria A, et al. Sonographie zur Untersuchung des Wirbelkanals bei Kälbern mit Neurologischen Symptomen. Klauentierpraxis 2014;22:125–30.
19. Gentile A, Testoni S, Franz S, et al. Spinal cord: ultrasonographic windows in calves. Lisbon (Portugal): Proceedings XXVII World Buiatrics Congress; 2012. p. 154.
20. Popesko P. Rind, junge Färse. Medianschnitt durch den Kopf. In: Popesko P, editor. Atlas der Topographischen Anatomie der Haustiere. Stuttgart (Germany): Enke Verlag; 2011. p. 30.
21. Stoffel MH. Meningen. In: Stoffel MH, editor. Funktionelle Neuroanatomie für die Tiermedizin. Stuttgart (Germany): Enke Verlag; 2011. p. 100–5.
22. König HE, Liebich HG, Červeny C. Nervensystem (Systema nervosum). In: König HE, Liebich HG, editors. Anatomie der Haussäugetiere: Lehrbuch und Farbatlas für Studium und Praxis. Stuttgart (Germany): Schattauer; 2005. p. 485–556.
23. Berg R, Müller K. Hals und Brustwand. In: Budras KD, Buda S, editors. Atlas der Anatomie des Rindes. Supplement: Klinisch-Funktionelle Anatomie. Hannover (Germany): Schlütersche Verlagsgesellschaft; 2007. p. 14–5.
24. Tucker RL. Ultrasound-guided biopsy. In: Rantanen RW, McKinnon AO, editors. Equine diagnostic ultrasonography. Baltimore (MD): Williams & Wilkins; 1998. p. 649–53.
25. Orrison WW, Eldevik OP, Sackett JF. Lateral C1-2 puncture for cervical myelography. Part III: historical, anatomic, and technical considerations. Radiology 1983; 146(2):401–8.
26. Patten BM. How much blood makes the cerebrospinal fluid bloody? J Am Med Assoc 1968;206(2):378.
27. Testoni S, Grandis A, Diana A, et al. Imaging diagnosis—ultrasonographic diagnosis of diplomyelia in a calf. Vet Radiol Ultrasound 2010;51(6):667–9.

Ultrasonography of the Tympanic Bullae and Larynx in Cattle

Véronique Bernier Gosselin, DVM, MSc[a], Marie Babkine, DVM, MSc[b], David Francoz, DVM, MSc[b],*

KEYWORDS

• Ultrasound • Middle ear • Otitis media • Arytenoid chondritis

KEY POINTS

• Ultrasonography of the tympanic bulla in calves is useful for the confirmation of middle ear infection in cases of clinical disease and for the detection of subclinical cases.

• Ultrasonography of the larynx may help with the diagnosis of laryngeal and pharyngeal diseases by providing information on nonluminal structures, such as laryngeal cartilages.

• Ultrasonography of these structures can be performed in the field using a high-frequency (7.5-MHz) probe on a standing animal by a trained ultrasonographer.

INTRODUCTION

Diseases of the tympanic bullae or the larynx are not numerous in cattle but can be challenging for veterinary practitioners in the field. In the presence of suggestive clinical signs, confirmation of the involvement of these structures may rely on radiography, CT, or endoscopy. Unfortunately, these imaging techniques are not easily available or are not available at all in the field. With the widespread development of portable ultrasonography units and their availability in the field, ultrasonography of these 2 anatomic structures provides new diagnostic tools for the veterinary practitioner in a hospital setting as well as in field conditions. Recently, different studies have been published on ultrasonography of the tympanic bullae in calves. Ultrasonography of the larynx has only been reported in a case report and not been formally

The authors have nothing to disclose.
[a] Department of Veterinary Medicine and Surgery, College of Veterinary Medicine, University of Missouri, 900 East Campus Drive, Columbia, MO 65211, USA; [b] Department of Clinical Sciences, Faculty of Veterinary Medicine, University of Montreal, 1500 Rue des Vétérinaires, C.P. 5000, Saint-Hyacinthe, Quebec J2S 7C6, Canada
* Corresponding author.
E-mail address: david.francoz@umontreal.ca

presented. In other species, however, such as horses and humans, laryngeal ultrasonography and its use for the diagnosis of laryngeal diseases is well documented.

This article first reviews the ultrasonography of the tympanic bullae and its use for the diagnosis of otitis media in calves. Second, the ultrasonography of the larynx is presented. For both of these structures, brief anatomic reminders are first performed. Then, the scanning techniques and normal images are described. Finally, abnormal images of specific conditions are presented.

ULTRASONOGRAPHY OF THE TYMPANIC BULLA

In cattle, the primary disease of the middle ear, which encompasses the tympanic bulla, is otitis media. It has been associated with drooping ear, ptosis, head tilt, and purulent aural discharge, and a large proportion of otitis media can be subclinical.[1] The prevalence of clinical disease is highly variable depending on the study population, and the estimated prevalence in 1 study of subclinical cases of otitis media was 49.7%.[1] The most commonly used imaging diagnostic tools for middle ear diseases include radiography and CT. With these 2 techniques, the most frequent abnormality associated with a diagnosis of otitis media in calves is increased soft tissue opacity in the tympanic bulla and osteolysis of the trabeculae (radiography only).[2] Studies on the ultrasonography of the tympanic bullae in calves have recently been published, and similarly the most frequent abnormality described was abnormal content caused by the accumulation of fluid or exudate in the tympanic bulla.[1] Although the entirety of the tympanic bulla cannot be assessed with ultrasonography, this technique may be the more readily available on farms.

Anatomy of the Tympanic Bulla

The ear is anatomically divided into external ear, middle ear, and internal ear. The tympanic bulla is the most ventral part of the middle ear.[3] In cattle, it is divided into multiple air cells by thin osseous trabeculae oriented perpendicularly to the bulla wall.[4] Ultrasonography of the tympanic bulla in calves has been described and is best performed with a lateral approach.[5] With that approach, the lateral wall of the tympanic bulla is covered by the digastric and the occipitohyoidian muscles. The most dorsal part of the tympanic bulla and the tympanic cavity are obscured by the external ear canal. The most ventral part of the bulla is covered by the stylohyoid bone, which runs caudally then rostrodorsally. It turns into the stylohyoid cartilage, which courses in a depression in the most rostral part of the lateral bulla wall, is lined rostrodorsally by the vaginal crest, and ends as it attaches on the stylohoid process of the temporal bone. The paracondylar process of the temporal bone lines the tympanic bulla caudodorsally (**Fig. 1**).

Technique

Ultrasonography can be performed both in the hospital and under field conditions with a portable ultrasound unit.[1] This represents an advantage over other diagnostic imaging techniques, such as CT, which is limited to referral centers, and radiography, for which portable units are available to practitioners but interpretation is difficult due to superimposition of cranial structures.[2] The low cost and accessibility of ultrasonography also make it possible to perform sequential examinations to monitor the progression over time.[6] A high-frequency (7.5–10 MHz), short linear (38-mm) probe is recommended.[1,5] High-frequency convex and linear (60-mm) probes were found to have a lower handling ability than a short linear probe. A linear rectal probe offers a lower-quality image[5]; however, it is a good alternative when a short linear probe is not available.

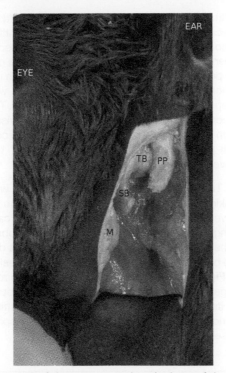

Fig. 1. Calf cadaver dissection of the area ventral to the base of the ear enclosing the tympanic bulla and landmarks from a lateral approach. M, caudal border of the mandible; PP, paracondylar process; SB, stylohyoid bone; TB, tympanic bulla.

Contention and preparation
The technique is well tolerated by calves and they can be restrained either standing or in sternal recumbency, without being sedated.[5] For screening purposes, both tympanic bullae of a calf can be performed without clipping within 5 minutes by an ultrasonographer acquainted with the technique.[7] The calf can have its head either straight or turned to one side, which may open up the space behind the mandible of the opposite side and allow for better contact and handling ability with the probe.[7] The hair below the base of the ear can be clipped for better contact.

Positioning of the probe
The probe is positioned just ventral to the base of the ear and caudal to the mandible. In previous studies, 3 positions were used, 1 allowing evaluation of the bulla in a transverse section and 2 in a longitudinal view.[1,5] It is the authors' opinion, however, that there is not much gain of information by performing both longitudinal positions. Moreover, perfect positioning and identification of all described landmarks may be difficult in these positions, although abnormalities can still be observed without perfect positioning. One longitudinal position is necessary because it allows for better examination of the bulla than the transverse position. From a practical perspective, the technique can be performed using the transverse position followed by either of the longitudinal positions. To facilitate learning, performing the technique on a newborn calf (<12 h of age) is recommended, because of the decreased soft tissue thickness and because visualization of the trabeculae helps confirm identification of the bulla and adequate positioning (discussed later).

Transverse position Ultrasound evaluation of the tympanic bulla should begin with the transverse position because it is the easier to obtain and identification of the bulla is facilitated by recognition of the stylohyoid cartilage. The transducer is positioned in a rostrocaudal axis, perpendicular to the vertical ramus of the mandible (**Fig. 2**). The major landmark in this position is the stylohyoid cartilage, which is visible in transverse section as a hypoechoic round structure covering the bulla wall. The bulla wall is convex and forms a depression below the cartilage (see **Fig. 2**). The mandibular ramus (rostral) and the paracondylar process (caudal) may also be visible. The main disadvantage of this position is the limited view of the bulla and its content. From this position, the longitudinal position can be obtained after a 90° rotation of the probe while staying at the level of the cartilage.

Longitudinal position The transducer is in a dorsoventral axis, with the beam oriented perpendicular to the skin or mildly rostrally. The long axis of the bulla is visible and its wall is convex. It is covered in its rostral part by the stylohyoid cartilage in longitudinal view; therefore, the longitudinal view may or may not include observation of the cartilage (which distinguishes between the 2 longitudinal positions described previously). The landmarks are the paracondylar process or the vaginal crest dorsally and the stylohoid bone ventrally (**Fig. 3**). The occipitohyoidian muscle can also be observed. This position offers the longer window for evaluation of the bulla (approximately 2 cm) and better visualization of its content. The main disadvantage of this position is the difficulty for an inexperienced eye to identify the bulla and to confirm adequate positioning, due to the absence of a characteristic landmark.

Normal Images

The wall of a healthy bulla has a smooth echogenic surface, convex in longitudinal position and convex caudally and concave rostrally below the stylohyoid cartilage in transverse position. The healthy bulla is filled with air; therefore, the bone-gas interface creates a combination of reverberation and shadow beyond the wall (see **Figs. 2** and **3**).[5]

One exception to this is in mature bovine fetuses and calves less than 12 hours of age, whose tympanic bullae were found filled with fluid on ultrasonography.[5] The time period over which fluid is normally present in the tympanic bulla after birth has not been determined. The presence of fluid instead of gas allows the beam to penetrate

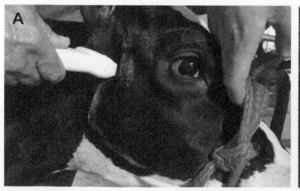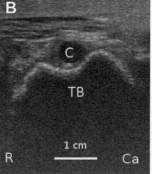

Fig. 2. Picture of the transverse position of the probe on a calf (*A*) and corresponding ultrasound image on a normal tympanic bulla (*B*). C, stylohyoid cartilage; Ca, caudal; R, rostral; TB, tympanic bulla.

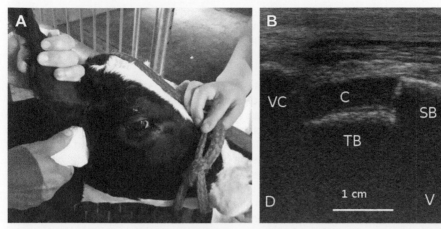

Fig. 3. Picture of the longitudinal position of the probe on a calf (*A*) and corresponding ultrasound image on a normal tympanic bulla (*B*). C, stylohyoid cartilage; D, dorsal; SB, stylohyoid bone; TB, tympanic bulla; V, ventral; VC, vaginal crest.

beyond the wall interface and reveal the content of the bulla. The resulting image is a smooth definition of the inner contour of the wall; trabeculae shown as thin hyperechoic lines spread like a fan in anechoic fluid (**Fig. 4**) and the medial wall in some cases. The presence of fluid and visualization of the trabeculae facilitated identification of the bulla in neonatal bovine cadavers,[5] and, in the authors' opinion, facilitates learning of the technique.

The technique has only been reportedly used in calves up to 10 weeks old.[5] In calves aged 19 to 50 days old, mean depth of the bulla (distance between skin and bulla wall) varied between age groups from 15 mm to 20 mm (Bernier Gosselin, unpublished data, 2013). Although it has not been evaluated in calves older than 10 weeks of age, it is possible that the increased depth of the bulla and increased thickness or

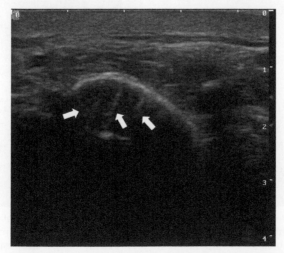

Fig. 4. Ultrasound image of a tympanic bulla of a neonatal bovine cadaver. Anechoic content and trabeculae, recognized as hyperechoic lines, are visible (*white arrows*).

ossification of the bulla wall affect image quality and evaluation of the bulla content.[5] With growth, changes in the anatomic structures surrounding the bulla may also affect the acoustic window and handling ability of the probe.

Abnormal Images

Ultrasonography of the tympanic bullae can be useful to detect pathologic changes that occur in the presence of otitis media. In the presence of clinical signs consistent with otitis media, ultrasonography can be useful to confirm diagnosis, define the extent of damage to the tympanic bulla, and evaluate the progression of lesions over time.[6] In the absence of clinical signs (drooping ear, ptosis, and head tilt), it can be used to detect subclinical otitis media, in research or in a clinical context on calves with unspecific fever and depression.[1,6] It can also be useful to estimate the prevalence of otitis media in a group, including subclinical cases.[1] Abnormalities reported in tympanic bullae affected with otitis media can be divided into content abnormalities and wall abnormalities. Content abnormalities include anechoic content with complete trabeculae, visible medial wall, mucosal edema, interrupted and irregular trabeculae, heterogeneous content, and abscessation[1,6] (**Fig. 5**).Wall abnormalities include irregular thickness, irregular contour, thinning, deformation, and rupture of the wall[1,6] (**Fig. 6**). In a study on mild to severe lesions of subclinical otitis media,[1] ultrasonographic abnormalities were often restricted to a portion of the bulla (**Fig. 7**). In these cases, it is important to scan the bulla thoroughly in longitudinal position while giving special attention to the most ventral part of the bulla. Content abnormalities were found more common and more indicative of early-stage of otitis than wall abnormalities. The presence of irregular or interrupted trabeculae was suggested to be more specific of pathology than intact trabeculae.

Diagnostic Value

Ultrasonography for the diagnosis of clinical and subclinical otitis media has been evaluated on calves aged 19 to 50 days old using histopathology as the gold

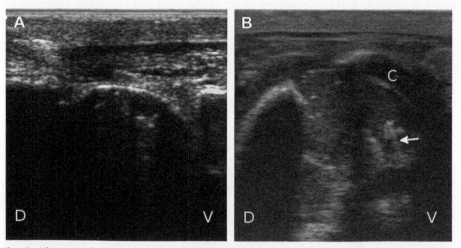

Fig. 5. Ultrasound images in longitudinal position of content abnormalities in tympanic bullae affected with otitis media. Variable amount of heterogeneous content can be seen (*A, B*), with trabeculae (*arrow* [*B*]). Image (*B*) illustrates that imperfect positioning and partial visualization of landmarks (eg, stylohyoid cartilage) does not prevent observation of abnormal content. C, stylohyoid cartilage; D, dorsal; V, ventral.

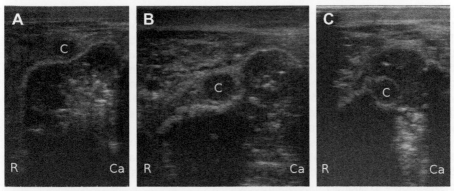

Fig. 6. Ultrasound images in transverse position of wall abnormalities in tympanic bullae affected with otitis media. Images show increasing severity of deformation (*A*, *B*) and rupture (*C*) of the caudal part of the bulla, associated with heterogeneous content. C, stylohyoid cartilage; Ca, caudal; R, rostral.

standard.[1] Two ultrasonographers performed the ultrasonography; one was more experienced than the other, although both were acquainted with the technique prior to the study. They classified the bullae as negative, suspicious (1 abnormality in <25% of the bulla in only 1 position), or positive (1 or more abnormalities in >25% of the bulla in 1 or more positions). On histopathology, 35 bullae were negative and 45 bullae were positive. Bullae that were positive on histopathology were further classified based on the detection of facial nerve deficits on neurologic examination: 16 bullae were clinically affected and 29 were subclinically affected. Depending on the ultrasonographer and the classification of suspicious bullae, sensitivity on all bullae

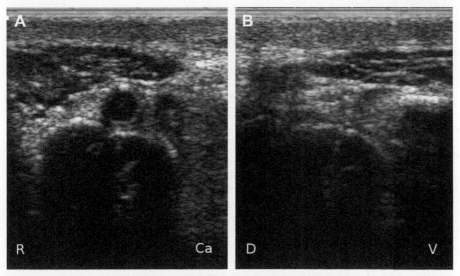

Fig. 7. Ultrasound images in transverse (*A*) and longitudinal (*B*) positions of tympanic bullae affected with otitis media. Abnormalities are limited to the caudal (*A*) or ventral (*B*) part of the bulla and consist in anechoic content with hyperechoic trabeculae (see **Fig. 4**). Ca, caudal; D, dorsal; R, rostral; V, ventral.

(clinical and subclinical) ranged from 36% to 63%. Sensitivity on subclinical bullae ranged from 23% to 55%, whereas it ranged from 56% to 94% on clinical bullae. The lower sensitivity in less severely affected bullae could be explained by the fact that visualization of the bulla content depends on the presence of exudate against the lateral wall (absence of bone-gas interface) in the acoustic window, and subtle changes can be confounded with artifacts. Despite a low sensitivity, ultrasonography was able to detect up to 55% of subclinically affected bullae, which would otherwise go undetected and untreated. Further studies are needed to evaluate the clinical relevance and benefit of treatment of subclinical otitis media.

Depending on the ultrasonographer and the classification of suspicious bullae, specificity ranged from 84% to 100%. Factors that could affect specificity include causes of nonpathologic accumulation of fluid in the bulla, as seen in newborn calves or secondary to auditory tube obstruction.

Agreement between 2 ultrasonographers acquainted with the technique was moderate ($\kappa = 0.53$). Intraobserver agreement between ultrasonography performed on the farm and in a hospital setting was also moderate ($\kappa = 0.48$). For the 2 ultrasonographers, agreement between real-time ultrasonography and re-reading of recorded images was moderate to substantial ($\kappa = 0.58$ and $\kappa = 0.75$, respectively).

ULTRASONOGRAPHY OF THE LARYNX

Diseases involving the larynx or pharynx are not common in cattle. They are often associated with problems of stridor, dysphagia, or dyspnea. Most often, these are pharyngeal or laryngeal, intraluminal or extraluminal masses, or abnormalities of the arytenoid cartilages.[8–10]

The complementary diagnostic tools most frequently used to specify the nature of the problem are radiography and endoscopy. These techniques allow the functioning of the larynx, the anatomy of the laryngeal and pharyngeal lumen, and the presence of masses distorting normal structures to be assessed. These tools do not provide information on nonluminal structures, such as laryngeal cartilages and muscles, and they are not always readily available.

In horses, ultrasound of the larynx has been studied several times, in particular in the diagnosis of arytenoid chondritis,[11,12] laryngeal dysplasia,[13] and laryngeal neuropathy[14,15] and during ultrasound-guided biopsy of the cricoarytenoideus lateralis muscle.[16]

In human medicine, laryngeal ultrasound is widely used for evaluation of the vocal cords and surrounding structures. Its minimally invasive character and the speed of execution make it a popular diagnostic tool.

Anatomy of the Larynx

The larynx is a hollow organ that controls the transit of air between the pharynx and the trachea.[17] It also contains the organs of phonation. Its rostral opening can be closed to protect the trachea and lungs, especially when swallowing.

It is composed of several cartilages covered with a mucosa on its inner surface. Cartilages are connected to one another and to the hyoid apparatus and the trachea by muscles and ligaments.

There are 5 main cartilages: 3 are odd and median—the cricoid, the thyroid, and the epiglottic, whereas the others are even—the arytenoid cartilages.

Muscles of interest during neurologic dysfunction are the cricoarytenoideus dorsalis and the cricoarytenoideus lateralis. The main structures are highlighted in **Fig. 8.**

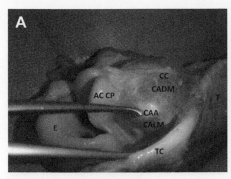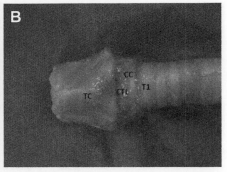

Fig. 8. Calf cadaver dissection of the larynx in dorsolateral view (A) and in ventral view (B). ACCP, arytenoid cartilage: corniculate process; CAA, cricoarytenoid joint; CADM, cricoarytenoideus dorsalis muscle; CALM, cricoarytenoideus lateralis muscle; CC, cricoid cartilage; CTL, cricothyroid ligament; E, epiglottis; T, trachea; T1, first ring of the trachea; TC, thyroid cartilage.

Technique and Normal Images

Ultrasonography can be performed both in hospital and under field conditions with a portable ultrasound unit using a high-frequency linear or sector transducer (minimum 7.5 MHz). The technique is well tolerated and can be performed on restrained animals. The hair of the larynx area can be clipped for better contact.

In horses, several acoustic windows (rostroventral, midventral, caudoventral, and caudolateral windows) have been described.[11] Anatomic differences between the 2 species, however, make some of these windows less interesting in cattle.

After manual palpation of the larynx, the probe is placed in longitudinal position relative to the calf at the caudoventral part of the larynx to see the cricoid cartilage just cranial to the trachea. The tracheal rings are easily recognizable. The cricothyroid ligament, which is tiny, is observed between the thyroid and cricoid cartilages (**Fig. 9**).

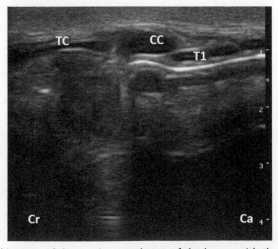

Fig. 9. Ultrasound images of the caudoventral part of the larynx with the probe in longitudinal position. Ca, caudal; CC, cricoid cartilage; Cr, cranial; TC, thyroid cartilage; T1, first ring of the trachea.

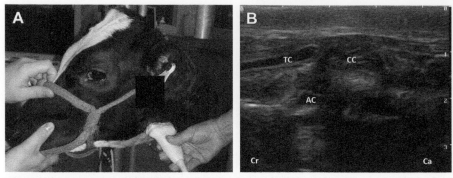

Fig. 10. Picture of the longitudinal position of the probe on a calf (*A*) and corresponding ultrasound image of the lateral part of the larynx (*B*). AC, arytenoid cartilage; Ca, caudal; CC, cricoid cartilage; Cr, cranial; TC, thyroid cartilage.

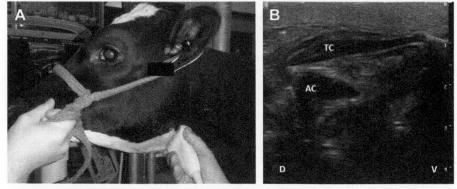

Fig. 11. Picture of the transverse position of the probe on a calf (*A*) and corresponding ultrasound image of the larynx (*B*). AC, arytenoid cartilage; D, dorsal; TC, thyroid cartilage; V, ventral.

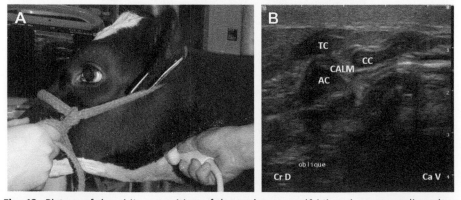

Fig. 12. Picture of the oblique position of the probe on a calf (*A*) and corresponding ultrasound image of the larynx (*B*). AC, arytenoid cartilage; CALM, cricoarytenoideus lateralis muscle; CaV, caudoventral; CC, cricoid cartilage; CrD, craniodorsal; TC, thyroid cartilage.

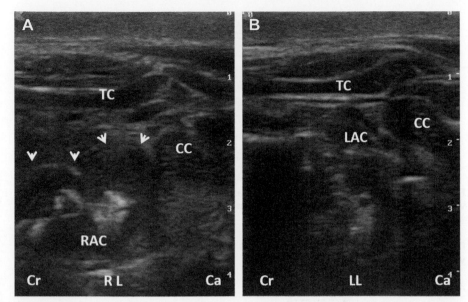

Fig. 13. Ultrasound images of a right arytenoid chondritis. Comparative images between the right (*A*) and left (*B*) arytenoid cartilages are presented. Ca, caudal; CC, cricoid cartilage; Cr, cranial; LAC, left arytenoid cartilage; LL, Left view of the larynx; RAC, right arytenoid cartilage; RL, Right view of the larynx; TC, thyroid cartilage. White arrows show the extended contour of the right arytenoid cartilage.

By moving the probe in the lateral part, while remaining in longitudinal position (**Fig. 10**), thyroid, arytenoid, and cricoid cartilages are visualized. The elongated shape of the thyroid cartilage makes it easily recognizable. This position allows only a small part of the arytenoid cartilage to be seen, but it is useful because it can identify this cartilage (see **Fig. 10**).

By rotating the probe in a transverse position (**Fig. 11**), a greater part of the arytenoid cartilage is highlighted (see **Fig. 11**).

An oblique position (**Fig. 12**) allows visualizing the arytenoid and cricoid cartilages, cricoarytenoid articulation, and crycoarytenoideus lateralis muscle (see **Fig. 12**). As in

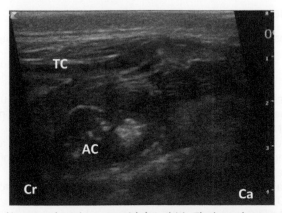

Fig. 14. Ultrasound images of a right arytenoid chondritis. The lateral aspect of the larynx is seen in longitudinal position. AC, arytenoid cartilage; Ca, caudal; Cr, cranial; TC, thyroid cartilage.

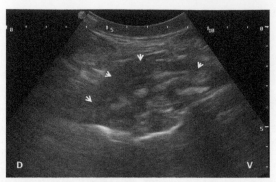

Fig. 15. Ultrasound image of tumoral infiltration of the arytenoid cartilage (lymphoma). White arrows mark the outline of the infiltrated arytenoid cartilage. D, dorsal; V, ventral.

horses, evaluation of this muscle could be considered in the case of laryngeal paralysis (size and biopsy).[15,16]

Abnormal Images and Diagnostic Value

As discussed previously, laryngeal diseases are not frequent and numerous in cattle. As a consequence, the diagnostic value of this complementary examination is not known. Ultrasonography of the larynx, however, can provide information on nonluminal structures, such as laryngeal cartilages. Additionally, it has advantages over radiography and endoscopy, 2 diagnostic tools that are frequently used in cases of laryngeal disorders, because it is more easily available in the field.

Laryngeal ultrasonography may be useful for the diagnosis of arytenoid chondritis. In such cases, the arytenoid cartilage may appear larger and deformed as well as heterogeneous with very hyperechoic areas (**Figs. 13** and **14**). Tumoral infiltration of the larynx (lymphoma) may also be suspected based on the images obtained on ultrasonography. At that time, the perilaryngeal tissues as well as laryngeal structures may appear heterogeneous (**Fig. 15**). Finally, the ultrasound recognition of normal laryngeal structures also allows a diagnosis of exclusion when it comes to perilaryngeal or pharyngeal masses.

ACKNOWLEDGMENTS

The authors thank ME Bilodeau for her help in the translation of part of the article.

REFERENCES

1. Bernier Gosselin V, Babkine M, Gains MJ, et al. Validation of an ultrasound imaging technique of the tympanic bullae for the diagnosis of otitis media in calves. J Vet Intern Med 2014;28(5):1594–601.
2. Finnen A, Blond L, Francoz D, et al. Comparison of computed tomography and routine radiography of the tympanic bullae in the diagnosis of otitis media in the calf. J Vet Intern Med 2011;25(1):143–7.
3. Dyce KM, Sack WO, Wensing CJG. Textbook of veterinary anatomy. 4th edition. St Louis (MO): Saunders/Elsevier; 2010.
4. Jensen R, Maki LR, Lauerman LH, et al. Cause and pathogenesis of middle ear infection in young feedlot cattle. J Am Vet Med Assoc 1983;182(9):967–72.

5. Bernier Gosselin V, Babkine M, Nichols S, et al. Ultrasound evaluation of tympanic bulla in calves. Can Vet J 2012;53(8):849–54.
6. Bernier Gosselin V, Francoz D, Babkine M, et al. A retrospective study of 29 cases of otitis media/interna in dairy calves. Can Vet J 2012;53(9):957–62.
7. Bernier Gosselin V. Validation of an ultrasound imaging technique of the tympanic bullae for the diagnosis of otitis media in calves [master's thesis]. Montréal (Canada): Université de Montréal; 2013 [in French].
8. Lardé H, Nichols S, Babkine M, et al. Laryngeal obstruction caused by lymphoma in an adult dairy cow. Can Vet J 2014;55(2):136–40.
9. Boileau MJ, Jann HW, Confer AW. Use of a chain écraseur for excision of a pharyngeal granuloma in a cow. J Am Vet Med Assoc 2009;234(7):935–7.
10. Nichols S, Anderson DE. Subtotal or partial unilateral arytenoidectomy for treatment of arytenoid chondritis in five calves. J Am Vet Med Assoc 2009;235(4):420–5.
11. Chalmers HJ, Cheetham J, Yeager AE, et al. Ultrasonography of the equine larynx. Vet Radiol Ultrasound 2006;47(5):476–81.
12. Garrett KS, Embertson RM, Woodie JB, et al. Ultrasound features of arytenoid chondritis in Thoroughbred horses. Equine Vet J 2013;45(5):598–603.
13. Garrett KS, Woodie JB, Embertson RM, et al. Diagnosis of laryngeal dysplasia in five horses using magnetic resonance imaging and ultrasonography. Equine Vet J 2009;41(8):766–71.
14. Chalmers HJ, Yeager AE, Cheetham J, et al. Diagnostic sensitivity of subjective and quantitative laryngeal ultrasonography for recurrent laryngeal neuropathy in horses. Vet Radiol Ultrasound 2012;53(6):660–6.
15. Chalmers HJ, Viel L, Caswell JL, et al. Ultrasonographic detection of early atrophy of the intrinsic laryngeal muscles of horses. Am J Vet Res 2015;76(5):426–36.
16. O'Neill HD, Ballegeer EA, De Feijter-Rupp HL, et al. Ultrasound-guided biopsy of the cricoarytenoideus lateralis muscle: technique and safety in horses. Equine Vet J 2014;46(2):244–8.
17. Barone R. Anatomie comparée des mammifères domestiques. Tome 3 splanchnologie 1. 3rd edition. Paris: Vigot; 1997.

Ultrasound-Guided Nerve Block Anesthesia

Michela Re, Dr Med Vet, Javier Blanco, Dr Med Vet,
Ignacio A. Gómez de Segura, Dr Med Vet*

KEYWORDS

- Cattle • Ultrasonography • Analgesia • Locoregional anesthesia • Nerve block

KEY POINTS

- Superficial nerves may be easily identifiable through ultrasonography in the cattle and facilitate local anesthetic disposition around nerve structures.
- Ultrasound-guided nerve block greatly increases the accuracy of local anesthetic administration around the nerve.
- Advantages may include an improved degree and duration of nerve blockade while reducing the dose of local anesthetic.
- Conduction nerves of clinical interest that may benefit from ultrasonography include the paravertebral nerves, the epidural space, the sciatic and femoral nerves for hind limb procedures, the brachial plexus for forelimb procedures, and the cornual, auriculoparpebral, and infraorbital nerves in the head.

INTRODUCTION

Local and regional anesthetic techniques are preferred methods of anesthesia in ruminants because they facilitate clinical work with the animal in the standing position, sedated or not, and are safe, inexpensive techniques, while providing analgesia with minimal adverse effects. Common locoregional anesthetic techniques include local infiltration and line block; paravertebral block; epidural anesthesia; and blockade of the foot, eye, or the horn among other techniques.[1] Anesthetic techniques based on nerve conduction block may be preferred compared with tissue infiltration when the painful anatomic area is infected, ischemic, or injured. When a blind nerve conduction block is produced the experience and skills of the clinician greatly influence the success rate. To improve it, ultrasound-guided techniques of local anesthesia are increasingly used in small animals.[2] Furthermore, in people the cost-effectiveness of ultrasound-guided

Disclosure Statement: The authors have nothing to disclose.
Department of Animal Medicine and Surgery, Veterinary Faculty, Complutense University of Madrid, Avda Puerta de Hierro s/n, Madrid 28040, Spain
* Corresponding author.
E-mail address: iagsegura@vet.ucm.es

regional anesthesia has been demonstrated.[3] Electrostimulation of targeted nerves is an alternative but also complementary technique to ultrasound-guided nerve localization.[4]

In ruminants only a few techniques have been studied with ultrasonography and further research is needed to determine the techniques of potential use in the future. Therefore, clinicians may anticipate the description of ultrasound-guidance for most techniques already performed blindly in the clinical setting and where a higher degree of success is desirable. New techniques may be developed, mostly based on previous work performed in small animals[2] and people.[5,6]

Regional anesthetic techniques require knowledge of the anatomic area to be desensitized. Disadvantages may include the difficulty in identifying anatomic landmarks, variability in anatomic pathways of peripheral nerves, risk of penetrating into other structures (eg, an accidental intraperitoneal administration instead of subcutaneous injection), or the large volume of local anesthetic. The variable anatomy between individuals may lead to poor success rates for specific peripheral nerve blocks.[7,8] Large volumes of local anesthetics are most likely administered to compensate for inaccurate needle placement within the blocked nerve. However, despite the large volumes used the success rate may also be lower than expected because of an inaccurate local anesthetic deposition relative to the nerve structures.[5] Side effects may be expected from large doses, especially when these drugs are combined with epinephrine.[7]

ULTRASOUND IN REGIONAL ANESTHESIA

Ultrasonography allows the identification of the neural structures and the adjacent anatomic structures, besides eventual anatomic variants. The use of an ultrasound device with multifrequency 5.0- to 7.5-MHz linear transducer in bovine reproduction may greatly facilitate its use to improve regional anesthetic techniques. Bovine clinicians may easily benefit from their expertise in the use of ultrasound devices by identifying nerve structures and improving local anesthetic administration accuracy and effectiveness. However, to achieve a wider use of ultrasound-guided nerve block experimental and clinical studies are required to describe the anatomic landmarks and identify suitable acoustic windows, but also the actual efficacy of these techniques compared with the standard blind anesthetic block.

Regional anesthetic techniques benefit from administering the drug in the right place with the lowest effective dose. This not only spares drug use but also increases the safety margin. Accuracy is largely favored by direct needle visualization together with the anatomic structures including the nerves. Visualization of anesthetic spreading further facilitates the overall process. Although epineural and subperineural or intrafascicular injections may also occur there is evidence, although controversial,[9,10] that the latter occurrence is relatively safe.[11]

The usefulness of ultrasound guidance for regional nerve block techniques includes the localization of anatomic structures and landmarks despite variability in anatomic pathways of peripheral nerves. Because of the visualization of the different anatomic structures the risk of penetrating adjacent tissues, such as vessels or internal organs, is largely reduced, as is the required volume of local anesthetic. However, despite improved accuracy with ultrasound guidance, the spread of the local anesthetic cannot be predicted and adjustments of the needle tip are recommended.[5]

ADVANTAGES OF ULTRASOUND GUIDANCE IN REGIONAL ANESTHESIA
Visualization of Anatomic Structures

Ultrasound guidance allows visualization of the neural and adjacent anatomic structures, including arteries, veins, pleura,[12] or internal organs, such as the rumen or kidneys. Tendons, nerves, and fascia typically appear as hyperechoic, whereas fat and muscle are seen as heterogeneous, hypoechoic structures. Fluids in arteries and veins appear as anechoic, whereas air is shown as a bright, hyperechoic image. Vessel identification prevents intravascular local anesthetic administration, whereas avoidance of fat tissue may avoid nerve block failure with the blind technique. High-frequency beams (10–15 MHz) improve the ability to distinguish between two structures in line with the beam (axial resolution), although limiting the depth of the visualized tissue.[13]

The gain, or the degree of amplification of ultrasound beams, should be adjusted so the background is mostly black and the nerves white (hyperechoic), and the opposite when the nerves are black.[14] The focus adjustment allows focusing the anatomic area of interest. Probe manipulation allows the application of pressure but also rotation, alignment, and tilt to better visualize the anatomic structures. For example, application of pressure allows distinguishing veins from arteries in close vicinity.

Reduction of Local Anesthetic Requirements

Direct local anesthetic spread visualization allows the use of a smaller volume of the drug while ensuring its correct disposition.[5] In people several studies have determined the minimum effective volumes for different regional blocks. This information is still lacking in cattle and is likely to allow a reduction of the total dose of local anesthetic required in this species. In the authors' experience, one-half of the dose/volume commonly used in the paravertebral nerve block produces at least a blockade similar to that obtained with the blind technique. However, a minimum effective dose is most probably only achieved by ultrasound-experienced clinicians and higher doses are likely required by most clinicians. In people, up to two to three times the minimum effective dose is required by less experienced clinicians.[5]

Improvement in Anesthetic Block Quality

The quality of the nerve block depends on several factors, including the local anesthetic used, its volume and concentration (dose), and the technique used to localize the nerve (blind, nerve stimulation, and ultrasound). In humans, ultrasound-guided blocks provide a faster onset time and longer duration compared with other nerve location techniques.[15–17]

Prevention of Fatalities

A maximum lidocaine dose of 10 mg/kg has been suggested in cattle to prevent toxicity,[1] which involves a large volume of 175 mL of lidocaine 2% in the 350-kg cattle. However, a sudden absorption of a smaller volume by its inadvertent administration into an artery or vein may produce acute toxicity. Visualization of great vessels with ultrasonography reduces the risk of vascular puncture.[18]

LOCALIZATION OF NERVES OF CLINICAL RELEVANCE

Direct visualization of nerves and adjacent anatomic structures is an obvious advantage of ultrasound-guided nerve block techniques. Blind landmark-guided approaches should theoretically provide a much lesser accuracy.[19]

Anatomy and Ultrasound Image of the Nerve

The ultrasound examination should start by identifying a known anatomic landmark near the nerve. Most peripheral nerves are visualized over their entire course. Their visibility is only limited where dorsal shadows of bone structures are present. The ultrasonographic image of the nerve varies from hypoechoic to hyperechoic depending on the quality of the ultrasound equipment, the size of the nerve, and the angle of the ultrasound beam. The nerve's image is sensitive to the angle of the beam, known as angle of insonation, because it contains and is often surrounded by fat.[14] A linear transducer is usually used to identify the nerves.

The nerve is localized in transverse scan, where the nerves appear as single or multiple round or oval hypoechoic areas encircled by a relatively hyperechoic horizon. The probe is then turned in the long axis of the nerve (longitudinal view) where the nerve is seen as a hyperechoic band characterized by multiple discontinuous hypoechoic stripes separated by hyperechoic lines (fascicle pattern).

These hyperechoic structures are the fascicles of the nerves, whereas the hypoechoic background reflects the connective tissue between neuronal structures. The nerve is more echogenic compared with the muscle, which shows hypoechoic muscle fiber bundles with intervening echogenic perimysium. The tendon is more echogenic compared with the nerve and shows a distinctive fibrillar pattern.[20]

Needle Visualization and Guidance

A main factor for successful nerve block is visualization of the needle together with the spread of local anesthetic during the injection, confirming the correct disposition of the local anesthetic around the nerve. Needle tip proximity to the nerve allows accurate disposition of the local anesthetic. However, common pitfalls include subfascial (muscular) administration of the drug preventing its administration around the nerve. In cattle an 18G 10- to 15-cm spinal needle is usually used for deeper nerves, such as the paravertebral or femoral nerves, whereas shorter needles are usually appropriate for more superficial nerves. Needle manufacturing technology has evolved to produce easily identifiable needles under ultrasound by creating a reflective texture in the surface of the needle.[21] However, these needles are not widely used and may increase the cost (Life-Tech Inc., TX, USA or Pajunk Medical Systems L.P, GA, USA).

Two approaches can be performed with the needle for any nerve block, known as in-plane or out-of-plane approaches. An in-plane approach is considered when the needle enters the skin at one side of the probe. The whole shaft of the needle is aligned with the ultrasound beam and visualized when advancing to the nerve. In the out-of-plane approach the needle enters the skin away from the probe toward it and only the needle tip is visualized (**Fig. 1**). Both approaches can be considered although the in-plane approach may further facilitate the technique. The sonolocation technique facilitates the visualization of the tip of the needle by injecting a small amount of local anesthetic.[14]

The Doughnut Sign

A full successful nerve blockade is thought to be the result of the blockade produced when the drug surrounds the full circumference of the nerve. This is easily recognized by identifying a hypoechoic band surrounding the hyperechoic nerve (doughnut sign). However, there is evidence that a full circumferential spread of the local anesthetic is not required to obtain a successful blockade.[22] Then a minimal volume should be considered.[23] The length of the nerve in contact with the anesthetic is also considered a major factor to achieve a successful block. In dogs a contact length of at least 2 cm has been considered evidence of successful block,[2] and in cattle a volume of 0.2 mL/kg of dye was enough to stain large nerves, such as the sciatic and femoral nerves, at least 2 cm.[24]

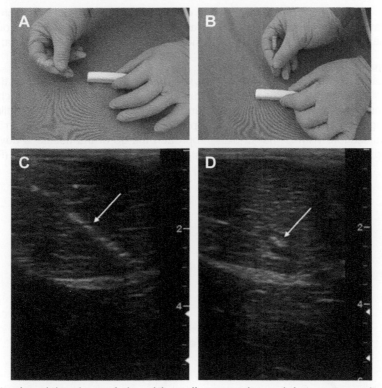

Fig. 1. In-plane (*A*) and out-of-plane (*B*) needle approaches and their corresponding ultrasound images. (*C* and *D*) Arrow indicates needle placement.

PERINEURAL BLOCK TECHNIQUES

Most commonly used blind regional anesthetic techniques have been described in detail elsewhere.[1,25]

Paravertebral Nerve Block

Paravertebral block produces analgesia of the flank area by typically blocking the nerves T13, L1, and L2.

Description

The proximal paravertebral block, where perineural injection is in proximity to the vertebral canal, may provide better clinical analgesia compared with the inverted L block for flank laparotomy in cattle.[26] The distal paravertebral block may also provide more consistent results, although larger doses of the local anesthetic are required with variations in efficiency because of anatomic variability of nerve pathways.[27] Ultrasound-guided needle placement for paravertebral nerve blockade has been described in cattle by identifying the articular processes of the vertebral segments with a 3.5-MHz curved linear array.[28] The transducer was placed parallel to the midline to visualize the articular processes to inject cranial and ventral to their most cranial aspects.[28] An in-plane approach for needle insertion was used and 20 mL was applied to T13, L1, and L2 (total of 60 mL). However, the paravertebral nerves were not identified, which may explain a poor anesthetic success rate similar to that obtained with the blind technique.[26] In the authors' experience, ultrasound guidance of the paravertebral nerves through direct visualization increases the overall success rate but also the onset, intensity, and duration of the paravertebral block compared with the blind technique (unpublished data, 2015).

Technique

Visualization of the paravertebral branches is obtained by placing the probe at the corresponding paravertebral space with the transducer placed in a lateral approach in the intertransverse space of T13-L1, L1-L2, and L2-L3 perpendicular to the midline. By localizing the distal part of the transverse process, the nerves are identified in its longitudinal section. With an out-of-plane approach the tip of the needle is advanced perpendicular to the skin plane at the distal part of the transverse process (**Fig. 2**).

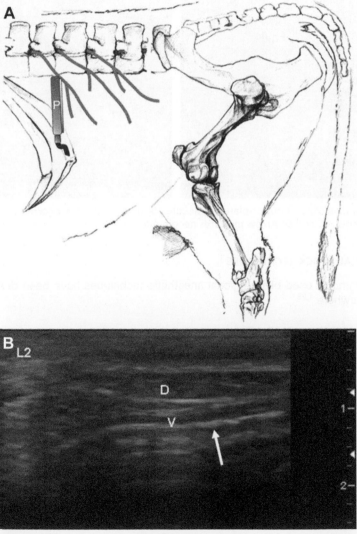

Fig. 2. Paravertebral nerve block probe placement (*A*) and the corresponding ultrasound image (*B*). D, dorsal branch; L2, transverse process of second lumbar vertebrae; V, ventral branch. Arrow indicates the ruminal wall.

Once the tip of the needle is within 1 to 2 mm from each nerve branch the local anesthetic is administered (10 mL per nerve).

Caudal Epidural Block

Caudal epidural administration of local anesthetics blocks nerves innervating the perineum and caudal surface of udder, skin over the semitendinosus and semimembranosus muscles, perineal muscles, scrotum, labia, vagina, vulva, prepuce, penis, and clitoris among other related structures.[25]

Description

Conditions where ultrasound guidance is of clinical benefit may include excessive body condition; fat accumulation at the tail base; exostosis or sacrococcygeal/intercoccygeal trauma, malformations, or fibrosis derived from previous trauma where identification of the epidural space is difficult. Also, the local anesthetic may be injected into fat and/or vessels. Failure of the technique may include subcutaneous or intravascular injection, or incomplete injection into the epidural space.[25] The sacrococcigeal space (S5–Co1 or Co1–Co2, high and low, respectively) is easily identifiable with ultrasonography and may facilitate proper needle insertion and drug administration. Also, a catheter may be advanced under direct visualization for intermittent administration of local anesthesia.

Technique

The ultrasound probe is placed perpendicular to the spine at the sacrococcygeal space where the full depth of the vertebral canal is visualized. The needle is inserted with an out-of-plane approach (**Fig. 3**).

Fore Limb Anesthesia: Brachial Plexus Block

Brachial plexus block produces analgesia and immobilization of the forelimb distal to and including the elbow by blocking C6, C7, C8, T1, and T2 nerves.[29]

Description

Brachial plexus block allows surgery under deep sedation and can be used under field conditions. Potential complications of the blind technique include pneumothorax and pyothorax[29] and vessel puncture.[1] This technique has been described experimentally in calves only,[18] which were administered lidocaine 2% (10 mL per nerve). The different nerves of the brachial plexus were not actually identified in this report and successful block was not achieved in all limbs. As an expected advantage, the brachial plexus was clearly differentiated from the axillary artery and vein branches minimizing the likelihood of intravascular injection.

Technique

Calves were positioned in lateral recumbency with the shoulder pulled caudally. To identify the brachial plexus the probe (4–10-MHz linear transducer) is placed on the first rib cranial to the acromion, which is used as the landmark for needle insertion with the blind technique.[30] The probe is first positioned transverse to the rib and then rotated 90° cranial to the first rib and moved dorsally to avoid displaying the large vessels and facilitate visualization of the brachial plexus. The needle is inserted with an in-plane approach dorsoventrally toward the brachial plexus cranial to the first rib, immediately ventral to the seventh cervical vertebra. The brachial plexus is visualized as multiple hypoechoic structures surrounded by a hyperechoic rim or band characterized by multiple discontinuous hypoechoic strips separated by hypoechoic lines (**Fig. 4**).[18]

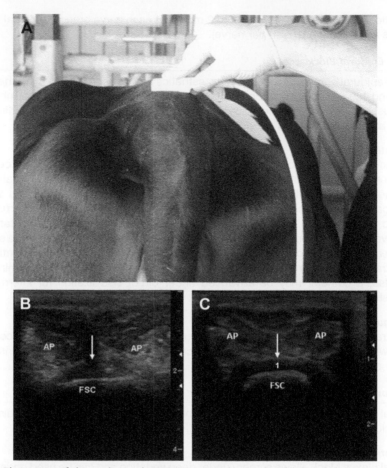

Fig. 3. Placement of the probe at the sacrococcygeal space level (*A*) and the corresponding ultrasound imaging of the epidural space in the cow (*B*) and calf (*C*). AP, articular process of the L1 vertebra; FSC, floor of the spinal canal, 1 shows the depth of the epidural space in the calf (0.2 mm). Arrow indicates the epidural space.

Hind Limb Anesthesia: Sciatic and Femoral Nerve Block

Unilateral block of the hind limb may be achieved by blockade of the two major nerves innervating it, the sciatic and femoral nerves.[24] These nerves blocks have been described in calves but not in the adult cow.

Sciatic Nerve Block

Anatomic area
The sciatic nerve innervates most of the lateral aspect of the hind limb and runs distal to the greater trochanter of the femur and caudal to the femoral shaft. The proximal third of the femur is the preferred anatomic area for sciatic block where the nerve runs alone and is easily accessed away from any other major nerve or vessel.

Description
By blocking the sciatic nerve in experimental calves,[24] complete analgesia has been observed in 6 out of 10 calves limbs. However, the medial subareas of the proximal

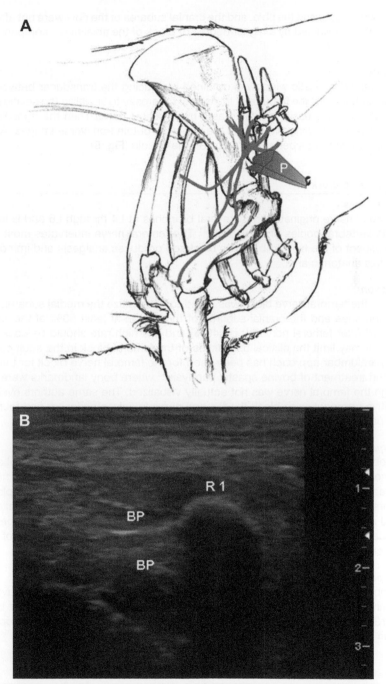

Fig. 4. Positioning of the ultrasound probe used to visualize the brachial plexus (*A*) and corresponding transverse ultrasound image (*B*). BP, brachial plexus; R 1, first rib.

metatarsus, tarsus, and the tibia, and the cranial subarea of the tibia were not affected. This might be explained by a higher degree of block of the tibial nerve compared with the peroneal nerve.

Technique

The suggested acoustic window is obtained by placing the transducer between the greater trochanter of the femur and the ischial tuberosity to visualize the sciatic nerve. The sciatic nerve is easily identified as a hyperechoic band. Then the transducer is moved distally, following the path of the nerve, to obtain transverse images. An out-of-plane approach has been used to guide the needle (**Fig. 5**).

Femoral Nerve Block

Anatomic area

The femoral nerve originates from several branches at L4 through L6 and is located near the vertebral bodies of L5 and L6.[31] The femoral nerve innervates most of the medial aspect of the hind limb and its blockade produces analgesia and immobilization of this anatomic area.

Description

In calves, the femoral nerve block was found to desensitize the medial subarea of the femur and knee and the cranial subarea of the tibia in at least 50% of the limbs.[24] Calves fell after femoral nerve block (40%) and this high rate should be considered because it may limit the clinical usefulness of the femoral block in the adult cattle. A dorsal paralumbar approach has been used for the femoral nerve block for the diagnosis and treatment of bovine spastic paralysis[32] where bony landmarks were used, although the femoral nerve was not actually visualized. The same authors evaluated alternative approaches to block the femoral nerve in calves cadavers and found the dorsal paravertebral approach to yield the best results.[31]

Technique: ilioventral approach

The probe is placed ventral to the wing of the ilium and along the longitudinal axis of the femoral nerve and rotated 90° to obtain transverse sections.[24] The femoral nerve is not as easily identifiable as the sciatic nerve and can be visualized in a cross-plane as a hyperechoic oval structure medial to the psoas major muscle and lateral to the femoral artery. The local anesthetic spreads directly in an anechoic space between the psoas major and iliacus muscles. The needle is inserted with an out-of-plane approach (**Fig. 6**).

Dorsal paravertebral approach

The probe is placed parallel to the spinal cord at the level of the sacrum and advanced in a cranial direction to identify the space between L5 and L6.[31] The probe is then rotated 90° and repositioned to visualize this space between the transverse processes of L5 an L6. The needle is inserted with an out-of-plane approach.

Anesthesia of Superficial Nerves of the Head

A description of the main nerves of the head of clinical relevance is found elsewhere.[25] Ultrasonography facilities visualization of nerves of the head in animals with thick skin where palpation is difficult. The cornual, auriculoparpebral, and infraorbital nerves are easily visualized, although there are yet no reports demonstrating the clinical advantages in cattle compared with the blind technique.

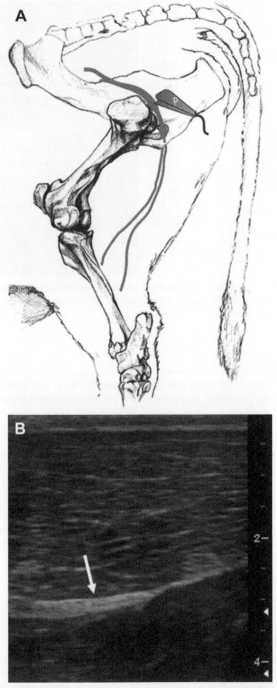

Fig. 5. Probe positioning for the visualization of the sciatic nerve (A) and corresponding transverse ultrasound image visualization of the sciatic nerve (B, arrow).

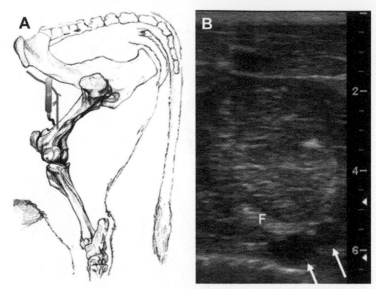

Fig. 6. Probe positioning for the visualization of the femoral nerve in calves (*A*) and corresponding transverse ultrasound image visualization (*B*). F, femoral nerve. Arrows indicate the femoral artery and vein.

Cornual Nerve Block

Main nerves innervating the horn are the cornual branch, the supraorbital, and the infratrochlear nerves. The latter two nerves are usually blocked by infiltrating the local anesthetic around the horn.

Technique
To block the cornual branch the probe is placed 2 to 3 cm medial to the zygomatic process perpendicular to the frontal line (**Fig. 7**A and D).

Auriculopalpebral Nerve Block

The auriculopalpebral nerve innervates the ear (rostral auricular branches) and the eyelids (zygomatic branches), facilitating eye examination by preventing blinking, although not providing sensory blockade.

Technique
The probe is placed caudolateral to the zygomatic process as shown in **Fig. 7**B and E.

Infraorbital Nerve Block

Infraorbital nerve block produces analgesia of the skin of the dorsal nasal area, nares, and upper lip and incomplete block of the nasal passages.[25] The infraorbital foramen is easily localized by palpation.

Technique
The probe is placed over the infraorbital foramen, which can be found 4 to 5 cm dorsal to the first molar on the maxilla (**Fig. 7**C and F).

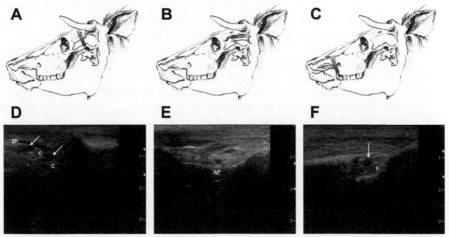

Fig. 7. Schematic view of the corneal (*A*), auriculoparpebral (*B*), and infraorbital (*C*) nerves with the suggested positioning of the probe and corresponding ultrasound image visualization (*D, E,* and *F,* respectively). AP, auriculoparpebral nerve; C, cornual nerve; I, infraorbital nerve; ZP, zygomatic process. Arrows indicate the cornual artery and vein in (*D*), and the infraorbital vein in (*F*).

COMPLICATIONS AND RISK

Ultrasound-guided nerve block should reduce the risk associated with locoregional anesthetic techniques as outlined previously. Intravascular, or other organ and tissues than nerves, injection is largely reduced. The dose required to produce successful anesthesia is also reduced thus decreasing the likelihood of overdose toxicity. Probably the main disadvantage of ultrasound-guided techniques is that more time is required to perform the technique and a minimum of experience with ultrasonography is required.

CURRENT CONTROVERSIES/FUTURE CONSIDERATIONS

Blind nerve block techniques are routinely and successfully used by bovine clinicians with noticeable experience. Therefore the use of ultrasonography might be considered unnecessary initially until sufficient knowledge is available demonstrating the advantages of this technique.[12] Ultrasound-guided nerve block is widely used in people and increasingly applied to small animals. Thus future experimental and clinical research in cattle should indicate which techniques would benefit from ultrasound-guided nerve block. In the authors' experience, these techniques may have a place in the clinical setting once the clinician has obtained experience with ultrasonography. Cheaper and handy ultrasound devices will help to spread the technique on farm. However, widespread use of these techniques will not be immediate.

REFERENCES

1. Anderson DE, Edmondson MA. Prevention and management of surgical pain in cattle. Vet Clin North Am Food Anim Pract 2013;29(1):157–84.
2. Campoy L, Bezuidenhout AJ, Gleed RD, et al. Ultrasound-guided approach for axillary brachial plexus, femoral nerve, and sciatic nerve blocks in dogs. Vet Anaesth Analg 2010;37(2):144–53.

3. Gonano C, Kettner SC, Ernstbrunner M, et al. Comparison of economical aspects of interscalene brachial plexus blockade and general anaesthesia for arthroscopic shoulder surgery. Br J Anaesth 2009;103(3):428–33.

4. Costa-Farre C, Blanch XS, Cruz JI, et al. Ultrasound guidance for the performance of sciatic and saphenous nerve blocks in dogs. Vet J 2011;187(2):221–4.

5. Marhofer P, Harrop-Griffiths W, Kettner SC, et al. Fifteen years of ultrasound guidance in regional anaesthesia: part 1. Br J Anaesth 2010;104(5):538–46.

6. Marhofer P, Harrop-Griffiths W, Willschke H, et al. Fifteen years of ultrasound guidance in regional anaesthesia: part 2-recent developments in block techniques. Br J Anaesth 2010;104(6):673–83.

7. Skarda RT. Local and regional anesthesia in ruminants and swine. Vet Clin North Am Food Anim Pract 1996;12(3):579–626.

8. Marhofer P, Willschke H, Kettner S. Current concepts and future trends in ultrasound-guided regional anesthesia. Curr Opin Anaesthesiol 2010;23(5):632–6.

9. Bigeleisen PE. Nerve puncture and apparent intraneural injection during ultrasound-guided axillary block does not invariably result in neurologic injury. Anesthesiology 2006;105(4):779–83.

10. Bigeleisen PE, Moayeri N, Groen GJ. Extraneural versus intraneural stimulation thresholds during ultrasound-guided supraclavicular block. Anesthesiology 2009;110(6):1235–43.

11. Belda E, Laredo FG, Gil F, et al. Ultrasound-guided administration of lidocaine into the sciatic nerve in a porcine model: correlation between the ultrasonographic evolution of the lesions, locomotor function and histological findings. Vet J 2014;200(1):170–4.

12. Denny NM, Harrop-Griffiths W. Location, location, location! Ultrasound imaging in regional anaesthesia. Br J Anaesth 2005;94(1):1–3.

13. Pollard BA. Ultrasound guidance for vascular access and regional anesthesia. Toronto: Library and archives Canada; 2012.

14. Bigeleisen PE, Orebaugh S. Principles of sonography. In: Kaye AD, Urman RD, Vadivelu N, editors. Essentials of regional anesthesia. New York: Springer-Verlag; 2012. p. 191–8.

15. Kapral S, Greher M, Huber G, et al. Ultrasonographic guidance improves the success rate of interscalene brachial plexus blockade. Reg Anesth Pain Med 2008;33(3):253–8.

16. Marhofer P, Sitzwohl C, Greher M, et al. Ultrasound guidance for infraclavicular brachial plexus anaesthesia in children. Anaesthesia 2004;59(7):642–6.

17. Oberndorfer U, Marhofer P, Bosenberg A, et al. Ultrasonographic guidance for sciatic and femoral nerve blocks in children. Br J Anaesth 2007;98(6):797–801.

18. Iwamoto J, Yamagishi N, Sasaki K, et al. A novel technique of ultrasound-guided brachial plexus block in calves. Res Vet Sci 2012;93(3):1467–71.

19. Weintraud M, Marhofer P, Bosenberg A, et al. Ilioinguinal/iliohypogastric blocks in children: where do we administer the local anesthetic without direct visualization? Anesth Analg 2008;106(1):89–93.

20. Suk JI, Walker FO, Cartwright MS. Ultrasound of peripheral nerves. Curr Neurol Neurosci Rep 2013;13(2):328.

21. Edgcombe H, Hocking G. Sonographic identification of needle tip by specialists and novices: a blinded comparison of 5 regional block needles in fresh human cadavers. Reg Anesth Pain Med 2010;35(2):207–11.

22. Kumar PAGB, Arora H. Ultrasound guidance in regional anaesthesia. J Anaesthesiol Clin Pharmacol 2007;23:8.

23. Latzke D, Marhofer P, Zeitlinger M, et al. Minimal local anaesthetic volumes for sciatic nerve block: evaluation of ED 99 in volunteers. Br J Anaesth 2010; 104(2):239–44.
24. Re M, Blanco-Murcia J, Villaescusa Fernandez A, et al. Ultrasound-guided anaesthetic blockade of the pelvic limb in calves. Vet J 2014;200(3):434–9.
25. Valverde A, Sinclair M. Ruminant and swine local anesthetic and analgesic techniques. In: Grimm K, Lamont L, Tranquilli W, et al, editors. Veterinary anesthesia and analgesia, the fifth edition of Lumb and Jones. 5th edition. Ames (IA): Wiley-Blackwell; 2015. p. 941–62.
26. Nuss K, Eiberle BJ, Sauter-Louis C. Comparison of two methods of local anaesthesia for laparotomy in cattle. Tierarztl Prax Ausg G Grosstiere Nutztiere 2012; 40(3):141–9.
27. Edwards B. Regional anaesthesia techniques in cattle. In Pract 2001;23(3): 142–9.
28. Kramer AH, Doherr MG, Stoffel MH, et al. Ultrasound-guided proximal paravertebral anaesthesia in cattle. Vet Anaesth Analg 2014;41(5):534–42.
29. Thurmon JC, Ko JCH. Anesthesia and chemical restraint. In: Greenough PR, Weaver AD, editors. Lameness in cattle. 3rd edition. Philadelphia: WB Saunders Co; 1997. p. 41–55.
30. Skarda RT, Tranquilli WJ. Local and regional anesthetic and analgesic techniques: ruminants and swine. In: Tranquilli WJ, Thurmon JC, Ko JCH, et al, editors. Lumb and Jones' veterinary anesthesia and analgesia. 4th edition. Ames (IA): Blackwell Publishing; 2007. p. 643–81.
31. De Vlamynck CA, Pille F, Hauspie S, et al. Evaluation of three approaches for performing ultrasonography-guided anesthetic blockade of the femoral nerve in calves. Am J Vet Res 2013;74(5):750–6.
32. De Vlamynck C, Vlaminck L, Hauspie S, et al. Ultrasound-guided femoral nerve block as a diagnostic aid in demonstrating quadriceps involvement in bovine spastic paresis. Vet J 2013;196(3):451–5.

Ultrasonographic Doppler Use for Female Reproduction Management

Heinrich Bollwein, PhD, DVM[a],*, Maike Heppelmann, DVM[b],
Johannes Lüttgenau, DVM[a]

KEYWORDS

- Doppler ultrasonography • Blood flow • Uterus • Ovary • Estrous cycle • Pregnancy
- Puerperium • Cattle

KEY POINTS

- During all reproductive stages, characteristic changes in uterine blood flow are observed.
- Within the first 3 weeks after insemination, before visibility of the embryo by B-mode sonography, differences in uterine and luteal blood supply are detected in early pregnant compared with cyclic cows.
- Because there is a high variability in uterine and in luteal blood flow these parameters are not useful for an early pregnancy diagnosis after a single investigation.
- Cows with puerperal disturbances show a delayed decrease in uterine blood flow in the first few weeks after parturition compared with healthy cows.
- Measurement of follicular blood flow may be used to identify normally developing follicles and to predict superovulatory response, whereas determination of luteal blood is a more reliable method than B-mode sonography to distinguish between functional and nonfunctional corpora lutea.

INTRODUCTION

The advent of B-mode ultrasonography in bovine reproduction in the 1980s heralded tremendous advances in research and clinical practice because it allowed for the first time the noninvasive visualization of the internal reproductive organs. Although organ morphology can be evaluated using this technique, it cannot provide information about organ function, such as vascular perfusion. Circulation of the bovine genital tract was initially investigated experimentally using invasive procedures.[1–3] For the

The authors have nothing to disclose.
[a] Clinic of Reproductive Medicine, Vetsuisse-Faculty, University of Zurich, Winterthurerstrasse 260, Zurich CH-8057, Switzerland; [b] Clinic for Cattle, University of Veterinary Medicine Hannover, Bischofsholer Damm 15, Hannover D-30173, Germany
* Corresponding author.
E-mail address: hbollwein@vetclinics.uzh.ch

past 15 years color Doppler ultrasonography has been increasingly used for blood flow studies in bovine reproduction.[4,5] This has led to new information about physiologic and pathologic processes of the genital tract in female cattle.

PRINCIPLE OF DOPPLER ULTRASONOGRAPHY

Ultrasound waves reflected from moving structures, such as red blood cells, differ in their frequency compared with the emitted waves, resulting in a Doppler shift. This shift is positive; that is, the frequency of the reflected waves is higher than that of the emitted waves when the red blood cells move toward the transducer. When the blood cells move away from the transducer, the frequency of the reflected waves is lower than that of the emitted waves and the Doppler shift becomes negative.[6]

TECHNIQUE OF DOPPLER ULTRASONOGRAPHY
Evaluation of Blood Flow

If the spectral mode of Doppler machines is used frequency shifts are displayed in a two-dimensional graph as a function of time, and a so-called Doppler wave is created in the course of the examination of the arterial blood flow during cardiac cycles (**Fig. 1**). In ultrasound machines with color Doppler capacity, the Doppler shifts are color-coded on the screen (**Fig. 2**). Positive shifts (blood flow toward the transducer) are usually indicated in red and negative shifts (blood flow away from the transducer) in blue. Power mode is an advanced method of imaging blood flow. In contrast to conventional methods, which measure the blood flow velocity, this technique measures blood flow intensity (ie, the number of red blood cells moving through a vessel per time unit). The blood cells are seen as colored foci projected onto the B-mode image. Compared with the conventional color Doppler technique, this method is superior for imaging very low blood flow, such as follicular blood flow (FBF) (**Fig. 3**).

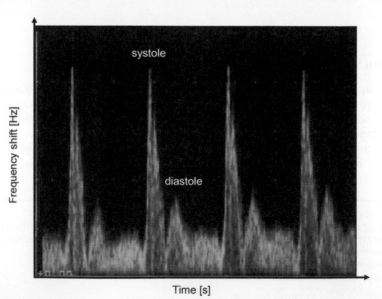

Fig. 1. Time-dependent changes in frequency shift of an artery during cardiac cycles detected by Doppler spectral mode.

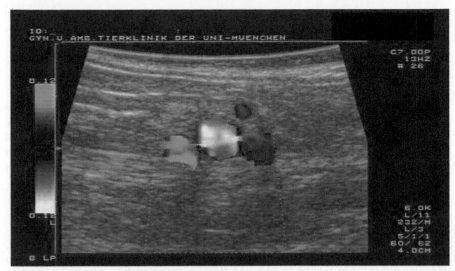

Fig. 2. Blood flow in vessels detected by color Doppler mode. Red shows blood flow moving toward the ultrasound probe and blue shows blood flow moving away from it.

Blood flow in individual vessels is typically evaluated semiquantitatively using the so-called Doppler indices (**Fig. 4**). These indices are not a direct measure of blood flow, but rather describe the resistance to blood flow in vessels peripheral to the vessel being examined. As the values increase, so does blood flow resistance and vice versa.[6] The Doppler indices are relative quantities obtained from the maximum systolic (S), minimum (M), end-diastolic (D), or time averaged mean frequency shift (TAMF) during one cardiac cycle (see **Fig. 3**). The so-called resistance index (RI) is calculated using the formula:

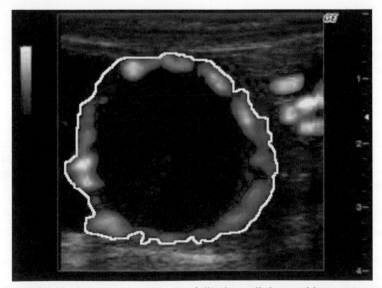

Fig. 3. Blood flow (*colored area*) within the follicular wall detected by power mode. The white line shows the borderline between the follicle and the ovarian tissue.

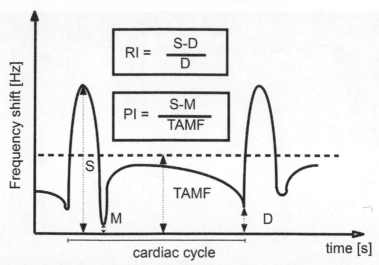

Fig. 4. Semiquantitative evaluation of blood flow by determination of the resistance to blood flow using the Doppler indices RI and PI. D, end diastolic frequency shift; M, minimum frequency shift; S, systolic frequency shift; TAMF, time averaged maximum frequency shift.

$$RI = (S-D)/S$$

However, differentiation of blood flow with an end-diastolic flow that goes to 0 is not possible using this index because, by definition, it assumes the maximum value of 1.[6] The pulsatility index (PI) is used to analyze this type of blood flow. The PI is used in tissues with a high vascular resistance, in which there is backflow of blood during diastole. The PI measures the total distance from the top to the bottom of the systolic peak and divides this by the mean velocity over the cardiac cycle. It is expressed as

$$PI = (S-M)/TAMF$$

S is the peak systolic frequency shift, M is the minimum diastolic frequency shift, and TAMF is the time averaged maximum frequency shift over the cardiac cycle.[6] For quantitative evaluation of blood flow, the blood flow volume (BFV) is calculated by using the time averaged maximum velocity and the area of cross-sectional area of the vessels (**Fig. 5**).

Because there are several blood vessels supplying the ovarian follicles and corpora lutea (CL), follicular and luteal blood flow (LBF) is most often not quantified by examining individual vessels, but by measuring the total area of colored pixels or the colored area in relation to the total area seen on cross-sectional B-mode images of these structures or in power mode (**Fig. 6**) using a computer-assisted image analysis software.[7]

Transrectal Localization of the Uterine Artery

To investigate blood flow in the uterine artery by using transrectal color Doppler sonography the aorta is first located (**Fig. 7**) and scanned in its caudal region to find the junction of the internal iliac artery. By following the latter distally, the branches of the rudimentary umbilical artery and the uterine artery are located. The uterine artery is the major blood vessel supplying the uterus and has a diameter of up to 5.0 mm in nonpregnant cows.[4]

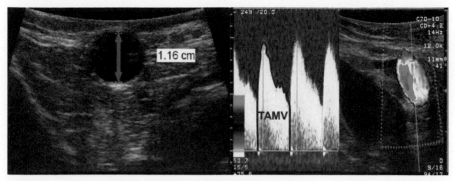

Fig. 5. Quantification of BFV flowing through a vessel. BFV (mL/min) = TAMV (cm/s) × 60 × π × D (cm²)/2; time averaged maximum velocity (TAMV) = TAMF × cos α; α = interrogation angle between Doppler beam and blood flow direction.

UTERINE BLOOD FLOW
Estrous Cycle

Uterine blood flow shows a characteristic pattern in cows (**Fig. 8**) with the highest time averaged maximum velocity values during proestrus and estrus. During diestrus, blood flow velocity remains at a fairly constant low level.[4] The cycle-associated changes in uterine blood flow velocity correlate with the plasma concentration of estrogens and progesterone (P4), although the correlations are only moderate. This finding indicates that not only sexual steroid hormones, but also other factors are involved in the regulation of uterine blood flow. However, these factors have not been identified.

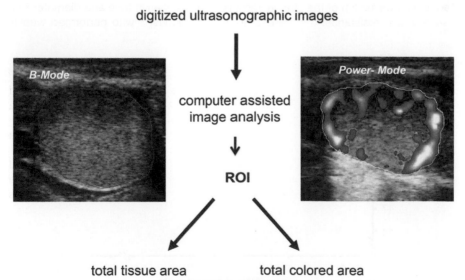

Fig. 6. Semiquantitative evaluation of blood perfusion on circumscribable tissues, such as the CL. The region of interest (ROI) on digitized ultrasonographic images is defined by the examiner and the total colored area or the colored area in relation to the total area of the tissue is measured by computer software.

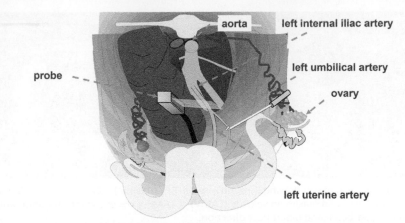

Fig. 7. Schematic presentation of the pelvic area of a cow and the position of the ultrasound transducer during Doppler sonographic examination of the uterine artery.

Pregnancy

In pregnant cows alterations in uterine blood supply are detected already within the first 3 weeks after insemination (**Fig. 9**). However, because there is a high variability in uterine blood flow not only within, but also between animals, it is not possible to diagnose early pregnancy by a single Doppler sonographic measurement of uterine blood flow. Similar to the estrous cycle the reasons for the changes in uterine blood flow during early pregnancy are not known up to now.[8]

Monthly evaluation of uterine perfusion during the whole pregnancy shows a strong increase of BFV. The RI decreases in the first 8 months of pregnancy and remains at a relatively constant level until calving.[9] The decrease in blood flow resistance is attributed to the conversion of the uterine vessels with changes in tone and diameter to a system of low resistance.[10-12] Panarace and colleagues,[13] who performed weekly

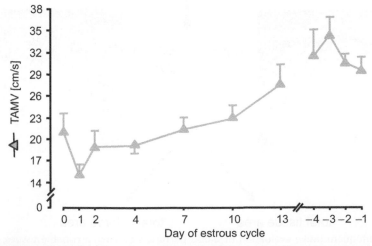

Fig. 8. Changes of uterine blood flow velocity (TAMV = time averaged maximum velocity) during the course of the estrous cycle in cows. Values are means ± standard error of the mean of four cows and two estrous cycles.

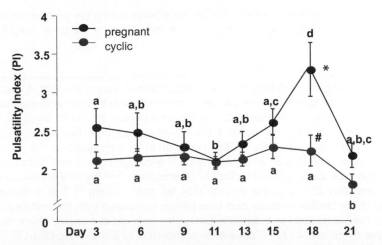

Fig. 9. Changes of resistance to blood in the periphery the uterine artery ipsilateral to the corpus luteum in cyclic (N = 14) and pregnant (N = 18) cows. Values with different letters differ (P<.05) within the same group of cows and values with different symbols (*, #) differ (P<.05) between groups of cows.

Doppler sonographic examinations of both uterine arteries during the whole pregnancy, observed between 22 and 26 weeks of pregnancy the disappearance of the notch, a protodiastolic incisure in the Doppler waves of the uterine artery. The authors suggested that this phenomenon could be used as an indicator of normal placental development, because in pregnant women the persistence of the notch during the last trimester is considered to be a sign for a deficient blood supply of the fetus.[14]

Because daily measurements of uterine blood flow during the last 7 days before parturition revealed no changes in BFV, it can be concluded that maximum blood flow capacity of the uterine arteries has been reached at this time. Birth weight of the calves was related to uterine perfusion at the end of pregnancy (**Fig. 10**).[15]

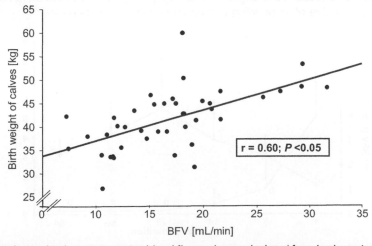

Fig. 10. Relationship between uterine blood flow volume calculated from both uterine arteries in week 39 of pregnancy and birth weight of calves. Values are from 42 cows and 42 calves.

Differences in the increase in BFV of the uterine arteries during the second half of pregnancy were more caused by the weight of the fetus than by the body weight of the cows.[16]

Puerperium

Alterations in uterine perfusion are most pronounced during the first 4 days after calving.[17] The changes in uterine perfusion coincide with the tremendous decrease in the size and weight of the uterus during this time period. In the course of the further puerperium the BFV decreases and the PI increased until Day 28 after calving (**Fig. 11**).[18] This is attributable to the completion of alterations in the caruncular vascular bed around Day 30 after parturition.[19] Although clinical and histologic uterine involution are accomplished by Day 47 postpartum,[19,20] the BFV showed a further decline until Day 65[21] and the PI until Day 86 after calving.[18] This indicates that changes of the uterine vascular bed take longer compared with the histologic alterations of the endometrium. A similar situation is observed in woman, where the highest PI was measured 40 to 50 days after completion of uterine involution.[22]

Puerperal uterine diseases like retained fetal membranes (RFM) and metritis have a negative impact on uterine involution.[23,24] Accordingly, uterine blood flow is also affected by puerperal uterine diseases. Cows with RFM show higher RI values of the uterine arteries already in the last days before calving, probably because of failure in the physiologic ablation process of the fetomaternal adherence.[15] On Day 8 after parturition cows with metritis have a higher BFV and lower PI values of the uterine arteries compared with healthy cows. The BFV in animals with uterine diseases exhibits no changes after Day 45 postpartum, whereas in healthy cows a further decline of the BFV occurs.[21] The altered blood flow parameters in cows with uterine diseases is interpreted as a reflection of a delayed uterine involution.

Besides the evaluation of uterine involution transrectal Doppler sonography can also be used for an indirect evaluation of uterine contractility. The arteries in the endometrium constrict proportionally to the magnitude of contraction followed by an increase of vascular resistance and a decrease of blood flow velocity in women.[25,26] Accordingly, in healthy cows an injection of oxytocin as a contractile agent on Day 2 after calving leads to a decline of BFV and an increase PI. Interestingly, animals with RFM showed no response to oxytocin challenge, suggesting that the uterus of these cows is not capable of responding to oxytocin during this time period.[27]

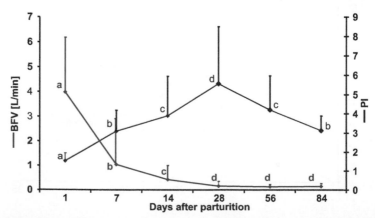

Fig. 11. Changes in uterine blood flow volume and pulsatility index of the uterine arteries during the first 12 weeks after parturition (N = 42). Values with different letters differ ($P<.05$).

OVARIAN BLOOD FLOW
Follicular Blood Flow

FBF has been examined by color Doppler ultrasonography during various stages of the estrous cycle. Small follicles (diameter >2.5 mm) with detectable blood flow 1 day before follicle selection subsequently develop larger diameters than those without detectable blood flow at this time.[28] An increase in FBF of the future dominant follicle (DF) occurs 1 or 2 days before diameter deviation.[29] After deviation, the probability[28,30] and the extent[31] of blood flow is higher in the DF compared with the second largest follicle. Although the difference in blood flow between the DF and the second largest follicle is supposed to be the result of follicular deviation but not to cause it,[31] blood supply seems to be essential for acquiring and maintaining follicular dominance.[30] Consistently, the major histologic characteristic of the dominant compared with the atretic follicle is its increased vascularity in the theca layer[32] that allows for enhanced delivery of gonadotropins and nutrients.[33–36] Results indicate that measurement of FBF is suitable to identify the future DF at an early developmental stage and to predict follicle viability after deviation. Furthermore, the examination of the number of follicles with detectable blood flow may be used to predict the superovulatory response.

During the periovulatory period, a functional relationship between FBF and plasma concentrations of estradiol (E2) and luteinizing hormone is described.[37] Before the luteinizing hormone surge, blood flow is detectable only in a small area in the base of the follicle, but FBF gradually increases in parallel with plasma E2 concentrations.[37] After the luteinizing hormone surge, there is a marked increase of blood flow to the base of the follicle, reaching its maximum before ovulation,[38] and a concomitant decrease of blood flow to the apex.[39] The increase in blood flow to the preovulatory follicle is supposed to increase the supply of gonadotropins and to facilitate the follicular rupture.[40] In contrast to the well-vascularized preovulatory follicles, atretic (anovulatory) follicles are characterized by a lack of detectable blood flow (**Fig. 12**).[37]

Therefore, measurements of FBF by color Doppler ultrasonography can be used to identify normally developing follicles and to predict the proximity of ovulation. The association between the presence of FBF and follicular E2 concentration is possibly due to E2 causing a rapid dilation of blood vessels by increasing the bioavailability of nitric oxide.[41] Consistently, the DF of the first ovarian follicular wave has not only a greater diameter and superior steroidogenesis than the DF of the second wave, but also a higher blood flow.[42]

Furthermore, color Doppler ultrasonography is advantageous compared with B-mode ultrasonography for differentiating follicular and luteal cysts, which is relevant to choose the appropriate treatment. The sensitivities of diagnosing luteinized follicles using B-mode (61.5%) and color Doppler ultrasonography (92.3%) indicate that blood flow more accurately reflects active luteal tissue than wall thickness.[43]

A positive relationship between the extent of blood flow of the preovulatory follicle at the time of artificial insemination (AI) and successful establishment of pregnancy is reported in cattle.[44] Although the mechanism for the reduced pregnancy rate in cows with lower FBF is not known, reduced mitochondrial oxidative phosphorylation in the oocytes may be involved.[44] In contrast, higher blood flow of the preovulatory follicle is associated with better *in vitro* cleavage rate of the recovered oocyte and subsequent embryo development.[45] Furthermore, Pancarci and colleagues[41] report the retrieval of better-quality cumulus oocyte complexes (COCs) from follicles with FBF compared with follicles without FBF, possibly because of a more estrogenic environment in the follicle or a better supply of nutritional and hormonal substances to COCs in follicular

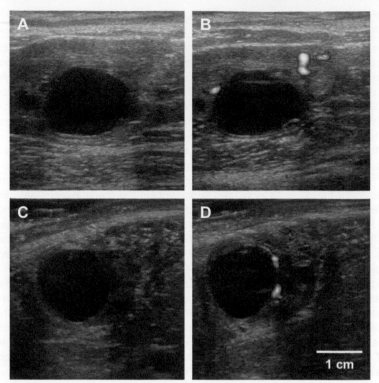

Fig. 12. B-mode (*A, C*) and color Doppler (*B, D*) sonograms of the bovine DF with maximum diameter on Day 8 of the estrous cycle (Day 1 = ovulation) before follicular atresia (*A, B*) and 36 hours before ovulation (*C, D*). Whereas the cross-sectional areas of the DFs are similar before atresia and ovulation, follicular blood flow is significantly higher in the preovulatory DF compared with the atretic (anovulatory) DF.

fluid. Therefore, the determination of FBF is a useful tool to predict the recovery of good quality COCs from cattle. Because the presence of FBF does not ensure the success of COC maturation, COCs obtained from follicles with FBF do not necessarily result in a higher chance of pregnancy.[41]

Vascular perfusion is higher in ovaries with a DF than in ovaries with neither DF nor CL, indicating an association between follicle growth and ovarian blood supply.[29] Furthermore, increased blood supply for the developing CL also increases the blood supply to the DF if the DF is in the same ovary, especially adjacent. Because one ovarian arterial branch supplies the DF and the CL when the two structures are in the same ovary,[29] luteal demands on blood supply have to be considered even for the assessment of FBF.

Luteal Blood Flow

Relating to the whole estrous cycle, correlation between LBF and P4 is higher than the correlations between the cross-sectional area of the CL (luteal size [LS]) and P4.[46] The close association between LBF and P4 is explainable because steroid precursors are provided to the CL via blood supply and the release of P4 into the circulation is also dependent on adequate LBF.[47]

In the early CL (Days 2–5), the blood flow gradually increases in parallel with the increase in luteal volume and plasma P4 concentrations, indicating active angiogenesis and normal luteal growth.[37] The developing CL becomes one of the most highly vascularized organs and receives the greatest rate of blood flow per unit of tissue for any organ of the body.[48] Because the increase in blood supply to the bovine CL is closely associated with enhanced plasma P4 concentrations, LBF seems to be a useful tool for assessing early luteal function. During the midluteal phase (Days 9–12), there are moderate and high positive correlations between luteal volume and P4 concentrations in plasma and luteal tissue, respectively.[49] Consistently, reduced luteal volume is associated with lower circulating P4 concentrations.[50] Therefore, the quantity of luteal cells seems to be decisive for the amount of P4 produced by the bovine CL. Because LBF and plasma P4 are closely related to the size of the CL, moderate positive correlations between LBF and P4 during the midluteal phase[46] probably result from LS instead from LBF. Using the relative LBF (quotient of LBF and LS) to exclude the influence of LS on LBF, no correlation between relative LBF and plasma P4 can be observed.[49] Therefore, the assessment of luteal P4 secretion by means of blood flow is not possible in the CL of the midluteal phase.

During the late luteal phase (Days 17 and 18), there is an initial increase in LBF in cows with spontaneous luteolysis, followed by a decrease 1 day later.[5] The decrease in LBF occurs in parallel with a decrease in P4,[51] and is followed by a decrease in LS 2 to 3 days afterward.[46] Functional luteolysis that is defined by decreasing P4 concentrations is already triggered by LBF, before a severe reduction of LS (structural luteolysis) can be observed. Although during the midluteal phase plasma P4 only correlates with LS but not with LBF, the functionality of the CL during the regression phase is better evaluated by LBF than by LS. Because of the close association between LBF and P4 during the early and late luteal stages, LBF can be used to distinguish between developing (functional) and regressing (nonfunctional) CLs of the same size (**Fig. 13**).

Because LBF decreases during the regression of the CL, it is supposed that monitoring of LBF can be used to diagnose early pregnancy in cattle. In a recent study,[52] cows have been artificially inseminated and retrospectively classified as pregnant (embryo with heart beat on Day 25 after estrus), nonpregnant (interestrus interval 15–21 days), or having an apparent embryonic loss (interestrus interval >25 days). On Day 15 after AI, which is a critical time for establishment of pregnancy in cattle,[53] LBF was significantly higher in pregnant cows than in nonpregnant or nonbred cows, indicating the different physiologic requirements of the CLs of pregnant and cyclic cows. Luteal regression in nonbred and nonpregnant cows is manifested by a significant reduction of LBF, LS, and plasma P4 on Day 18.[52] However, evaluation of LS by using B-mode ultrasonography does not allow a valid pregnancy diagnosis during the first 3 weeks of pregnancy because the functional regression of the CL precedes the morphologic regression. In contrast, assessment of LBF by using color Doppler ultrasonography improves the diagnosis of early pregnancy on Days 19 to 21 after insemination[38] because LBF reflects the functionality of the CL during the late luteal phase more reliably than LS.[28,46] Consistently, LBF clearly decreases at 19 days after ovulation in nonpregnant cows, but is continuously observed on Days 16 to 23 after ovulation in pregnant cows.[38] Although measurement of LBF is found to be more suitable for identifying nonpregnant than pregnant cows, it has not proved to be a reliable diagnostic tool for early pregnancy diagnosis mainly because of insufficient specificity.[54] However, in a recent study,[55] high sensitivity and a minimal percentage of false-negatives were found during pregnancy diagnosis at 20 days after AI using color Doppler ultrasonography in a large number of cows. In conclusion, LBF on Days 19 to 21 of early pregnancy is higher in pregnant than in

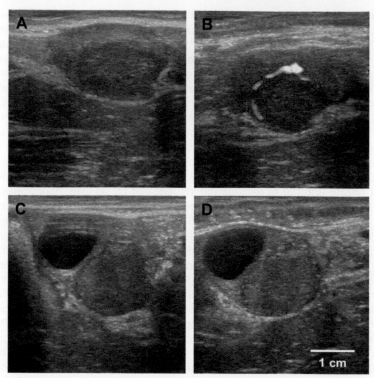

Fig. 13. B-mode (*A, C*) and color Doppler (*B, D*) sonograms of the bovine CL on Days 4 (*A, B*; Day 1 = ovulation) and 18 (*C, D*) of the estrous cycle. Whereas the cross-sectional areas of the CLs are similar in the early and late luteal phase, luteal blood flow is significantly higher in the developing CL compared with the regressing CL.

nonpregnant cows, and its assessment enables the early detection of nonpregnant cattle.

The LBF of cows with embryonic loss is similar to that of pregnant cows until Day 13 after estrus and does not increase thereafter, whereas the LBF of pregnant cows increases further on, probably because of the signaling of the conceptus.[52] In contrast, plasma P4 concentrations do not differ between pregnant cows and those with embryonic loss until Day 18 after estrus, indicating that LBF may be a more sensitive parameter regarding embryonic loss than plasma P4. From Days 25 to 40, luteal regression is detected at least 3 days after the detection of embryonic death.[56] Therefore, reduced LBF in cows during the third week after estrus may indicate subsequent embryonic loss, but LBF cannot be used for an early detection of future embryonic death from Day 25 onward.

SUMMARY

Studies performed during the last 15 years show that transrectal color Doppler ultrasonography is a useful technique for the noninvasive evaluation of genital perfusion in cattle. Determination of uterine and ovarian blood flow increases the knowledge about the physiology and pathophysiology of the reproductive tract of the cows. It is hoped that this information leads to improvements in the diagnosis and treatment of reproductive disorders in cows.

REFERENCES

1. Ford SP, Chenault JR, Echternkamp SE. Uterine blood flow of cows during the oestrous cycle and early pregnancy: effect of the conceptus on the uterine blood supply. J Reprod Fertil 1979;56:53–62.
2. Ford SP, Chenault JR. Blood flow to the corpus luteum-bearing ovary and ipsilateral uterine horn of cows during the oestrous cycle and early pregnancy. J Reprod Fertil 1981;62:555–62.
3. Ford SP. Maternal recognition of pregnancy in the ewe, cow and sow: vascular and immunological aspects. Theriogenology 1985;23:145–59.
4. Bollwein H, Meyer HH, Maierl J, et al. Transrectal Doppler sonography of uterine blood flow in cows during the estrous cycle. Theriogenology 2000;53: 1541–52.
5. Miyamoto A, Shirasuna K, Wijayagunawardane MPB, et al. Blood flow: a key regulatory component of corpus luteum function in the cow. Domest Anim Endocrinol 2005;29:329–39.
6. Dickey RP. Doppler ultrasound investigation of uterine and ovarian blood flow in infertility and early pregnancy. Hum Reprod Update 1997;3:467–503.
7. Herzog K, Bollwein H. Application of Doppler ultrasonography in cattle reproduction. Reprod Domest Anim 2007;42(Suppl 2):51–8.
8. Honnens A, Voss C, Herzog K, et al. Uterine blood flow during the first 3 weeks of pregnancy in dairy cows. Theriogenology 2008;70:1048–56.
9. Bollwein H, Baumgartner U, Stolla R. Transrectal Doppler sonography of uterine blood flow in cows during pregnancy. Theriogenology 2002;57:2053–61.
10. Deutinger J. Physiology of Doppler blood flow in maternal blood vessels in pregnancy. Gynäkologe 1992;25:284–91.
11. Gibbons GH, Dzau VJ. The emerging concept of vascular remodeling. N Engl J Med 1994;330:1431–8.
12. Starzyk KA, Pijnenborg R, Salafia CM. Decidual and vascular pathophysiology in pregnancy compromise. Semin Reprod Endocrinol 1999;17:63–72.
13. Panarace M, Garnil C, Marfil M, et al. Transrectal Doppler sonography for evaluation of uterine blood flow throughout pregnancy in 13 cows. Theriogenology 2006;66:2113–9.
14. Harrington K, Cooper D, Lees C, et al. Doppler ultrasound of the uterine arteries: the importance of bilateral notching in the prediction of pre-eclampsia, placental abruption or delivery of a small-for-gestational-age baby. Ultrasound Obstet Gynecol 1996;7:182–8.
15. Hartmann D, Honnens A, Piechotta M, et al. Effects of a protracted induction of parturition on the incidence of retained placenta and assessment of uterine artery blood flow as a measure of placental maturation in cattle. Theriogenology 2013; 80:176–84.
16. Herzog K, Koerte J, Flachowsky G, et al. Variability of uterine blood flow in lactating cows during the second half of gestation. Theriogenology 2011;75:1688–94.
17. Heppelmann M, Krüger L, Leidl S, et al. Transrectal Doppler sonography of uterine blood flow during the first two weeks after parturition in Simmenthal heifers. J Vet Sci 2013;14:323–7.
18. Krüger L, Koerte J, Tsousis G, et al. Transrectal Doppler sonography of uterine blood flow during the first 12 weeks after parturition in healthy dairy cows. Anim Reprod Sci 2009;114:23–31.
19. Gier HT, Marion GB. Uterus of cow after parturition: involutional changes. Am J Vet Res 1968;29:83–96.

20. Van Camp SD. Understanding the process of placental separation and uterine involution. Vet Med 1991;642–6.
21. Heppelmann M, Weinert M, Brömmling A, et al. The effect of puerperal uterine disease on uterine involution in cows assessed by Doppler sonography of the uterine arteries. Anim Reprod Sci 2014;143:1–7.
22. Tekay A, Jouppila P. A longitudinal Doppler ultrasonographic assessment of the alterations in peripheral vascular resistance of uterine arteries and ultrasonographic findings of the involuting uterus during the puerperium. Am J Obstet Gynecol 1993;168:190–8.
23. Fonseca FA, Britt JH, McDaniel BT, et al. Reproductive traits of Holsteins and Jerseys. Effects of age, milk yield, and clinical abnormalities on involution of cervix and uterus, ovulation, estrous cycles, detection of estrus, conception rate, and days open. J Dairy Sci 1983;66:1128–47.
24. Mateus L, da Costa LL, Bernardo F, et al. Influence of puerperal uterine infection on uterine involution and postpartum ovarian activity in dairy cows. Reprod Domest Anim 2002;37:31–5.
25. Fleischer A, Anyaegbunam AA, Schulman H, et al. Uterine and umbilical artery velocimetry during normal labor. Am J Obstet Gynecol 1987;157:40–3.
26. Janbu T, Nesheim BI. Uterine artery blood velocities during contractions in pregnancy and labour related to intrauterine pressure. Br J Obstet Gynaecol 1987;94:1150–5.
27. Magata F, Hartmann D, Ishii M, et al. Effects of exogenous oxytocin on uterine blood flow in puerperal dairy cows: the impact of days after parturition and retained fetal membranes. Vet J 2013;196:76–80.
28. Miyamoto A, Shirasuna K, Hayashi KG, et al. A potential use of color ultrasound as a tool for reproductive management: new observations using color ultrasound scanning that were not possible with Imaging only in black and white. J Reprod Dev 2006;52:153–60.
29. Ginther OJ, Rakesh HB, Hoffman MM. Blood flow to follicles and CL during development of the periovulatory follicular wave in heifers. Theriogenology 2014;82:304–11.
30. Acosta TJ, Hayashi KG, Matsui M, et al. Changes in follicular vascularity during the first follicular wave in lactating cows. J Reprod Dev 2005;51:273–80.
31. Pancarci SM, Güngör Ö, Atakisi O, et al. Changes in follicular blood flow and nitric oxide levels in follicular fluid during follicular deviation in cows. Anim Reprod Sci 2011;123:149–56.
32. Jiang JY, Macchiarelli G, Tsang BK, et al. Capillary angiogenesis and degeneration in bovine ovarian antral follicles. Reproduction 2003;125:211–23.
33. Zeleznik AJ, Schuler HM, Reichert LE. Gonadotropin-binding sites in the rhesus-monkey ovary: role of the vasculature in the selective distribution of human chorionic-gonadotropin to the preovulatory follicle. Endocrinology 1981;109:356–62.
34. Berisha B, Schams D, Kosmann M, et al. Expression and localisation of vascular endothelial growth factor and basic fibroblast growth factor during the final growth of bovine ovarian follicles. J Endocrinol 2000;167:371–82.
35. Zimmermann RC, Xiao E, Husami N, et al. Short-term administration of antivascular endothelial growth factor antibody in the late follicular phase delays follicular development in the rhesus monkey. J Clin Endocrinol Metab 2001;86:768–72.
36. Zimmermann RC, Xiao EN, Bohlen P, et al. Administration of antivascular endothelial growth factor receptor 2 antibody in the early follicular phase delays follicular selection and development in the rhesus monkey. Endocrinology 2002;143:2496–502.

37. Acosta TJ, Hayashi KG, Ohtani M, et al. Local changes in blood flow within the preovulatory follicle wall and early corpus luteum in cows. Reproduction 2003; 125:759–67.
38. Matsui M, Miyamoto A. Evaluation of ovarian blood flow by colour Doppler ultrasound: practical use for reproductive management in the cow. Vet J 2009;181: 232–40.
39. Brannstrom M, Zackrisson U, Hagstrom HG, et al. Preovulatory changes of blood flow in different regions of the human follicle. Fertil Steril 1998;69:435–42.
40. Acosta TJ. Studies of follicular vascularity associated with follicle selection and ovulation in cattle. J Reprod Dev 2007;53:39–44.
41. Pancarci SM, Ari UC, Atakisi O, et al. Nitric oxide concentrations, estradiol-17 beta progesterone ratio in follicular fluid, and COC quality with respect to perifollicular blood flow in cows. Anim Reprod Sci 2012;130:9–15.
42. Miura R, Haneda S, Lee HH, et al. Evidence that the dominant follicle of the first wave is more active than that of the second wave in terms of its growth rate, blood flow supply and steroidogenic capacity in cows. Anim Reprod Sci 2014;145: 114–22.
43. Rauch A, Kruger L, Miyamoto A, et al. Colour Doppler sonography of cystic ovarian follicles in cows. J Reprod Dev 2008;54:447–53.
44. Siddiqui MAR, Almamun M, Ginther OJ. Blood flow in the wall of the preovulatory follicle and its relationship to pregnancy establishment in heifers. Anim Reprod Sci 2009;113:287–92.
45. Siddiqui MAR, Gastal EL, Gastal MO, et al. Relationship of vascular perfusion of the wall of the preovulatory follicle to in vitro fertilisation and embryo development in heifers. Reproduction 2009;137:689–97.
46. Herzog K, Brockhan-Ludemann M, Kaske M, et al. Luteal blood flow is a more appropriate indicator for luteal function during the bovine estrous cycle than luteal size. Theriogenology 2010;73:691–7.
47. Janson PO, Damber JE, Axen C. Luteal blood-flow and progesterone secretion in pseudopregnant rabbits. J Reprod Fertil 1981;63:491–7.
48. Wiltbank MC, Dysko RC, Gallagher KP, et al. Relationship between blood-flow and steroidogenesis in the rabbit corpus-luteum. J Reprod Fertil 1988;84:513–20.
49. Lüttgenau J, Ulbrich SE, Beindorff N, et al. Plasma progesterone concentrations in the mid-luteal phase are dependent on luteal size, but independent of luteal blood flow and gene expression in lactating dairy cows. Anim Reprod Sci 2011;125:20–9.
50. Vasconcelos JLM, Sartori R, Oliveira HN, et al. Reduction in size of the ovulatory follicle reduces subsequent luteal size and pregnancy rate. Theriogenology 2001;56:307–14.
51. Shirasuna K, Asaoka H, Acosta TJ, et al. Endothelin-1 within the corpus luteum during spontaneous luteolysis in the cow: local interaction with prostaglandin F-2 alpha and angiotensin II. J Cardiovasc Pharmacol 2004;44:S252–5.
52. Herzog K, Voss C, Kastelic JP, et al. Luteal blood flow increases during the first three weeks of pregnancy in lactating dairy cows. Theriogenology 2011;75: 549–54.
53. Mann GE, Lamming GE, Robinson RS, et al. The regulation of interferon-tau production and uterine hormone receptors during early pregnancy. J Reprod Fertil 1999;54:317–28.
54. Utt MD, Johnson GL, Beal WE. The evaluation of corpus luteum blood flow using color-flow Doppler ultrasound for early pregnancy diagnosis in bovine embryo recipients. Theriogenology 2009;71:707–15.

55. Siqueira LGB, Areas VS, Ghetti AM, et al. Color Doppler flow imaging for the early detection of nonpregnant cattle at 20 days after timed artificial insemination. J Dairy Sci 2013;96:6461–72.
56. Kastelic JP, Bergfelt DR, Ginther OJ. Ultrasonic-detection of the conceptus and characterization of intrauterine fluid on days 10 to 22 in heifers. Theriogenology 1991;35:569–81.

Methods for and Implementation of Pregnancy Diagnosis in Dairy Cows

 CrossMark

Paul M. Fricke, PhD[a],*, Alessandro Ricci, DVM[b],
Julio O. Giordano, PhD[c], Paulo D. Carvalho, MS[a]

KEYWORDS

- Transrectal palpation • Transrectal ultrasonography • Pregnancy loss
- Progesterone • Pregnancy-associated glycoproteins

KEY POINTS

- Although coupling a nonpregnancy diagnosis with a management strategy to quickly re-initiate artificial insemination (AI) may improve reproductive efficiency by decreasing the interval between AI services, early pregnancy loss limits the accuracy of many direct and indirect methods for early pregnancy diagnosis currently under development.

- These limitations make the benefits of many currently available methods for early pregnancy diagnosis questionable and require that all cows diagnosed pregnant early after insemination be scheduled for pregnancy reconfirmations at later times during gestation to identify cows experiencing pregnancy loss.

- Although research and development efforts are being made toward development of an indirect pregnancy test for dairy cows, it remains to be seen whether these indirect tests will replace transrectal palpation or transrectal ultrasonography as the primary methods used for pregnancy diagnosis in dairy cows or whether veterinarians will combine these methods in a reproductive management program.

- Future technologies for pregnancy diagnosis in dairy cows may someday overcome current limitations of direct and indirect methods for pregnancy diagnosis, thereby improving reproductive performance.

The authors have nothing to disclose.
[a] Department of Dairy Science, University of Wisconsin-Madison, 1675 Observatory Drive, Madison, WI 53706, USA; [b] Department of Veterinary Science, University of Torino, Via Verdi, 8, Grugliasco 10090, Italy; [c] Department of Animal Science, Cornell University, 149 Morrison Hall, Ithaca, NY 14853, USA
* Corresponding author. Department of Dairy Science, University of Wisconsin-Madison, 1675 Observatory Drive, Madison, WI 53706, USA.
E-mail address: pmfricke@wisc.edu

ATTRIBUTES OF THE IDEAL PREGNANCY TEST

An ideal early pregnancy test for dairy cows would fulfill the following criteria:

1. High sensitivity (ie, correctly identify pregnant animals)
2. High specificity (ie, correctly identify nonpregnant animals)
3. Inexpensive to conduct
4. Simple to conduct under field conditions
5. Ability to determine pregnancy status at the time the test is performed

A final attribute of an ideal early pregnancy test would be the ability to determine pregnancy status without the need to physically handle the cow to conduct the test. Such a test may overcome the inherent limitations of current tests caused by pregnancy loss and may make pregnancy diagnosis before 28 to 35 days postpartum in dairy cows an economically viable reproductive management strategy. Although all of the methods described in this article require physical handling of individual cows to administer the test, future technologies for early pregnancy diagnosis may someday realize all of these criteria.

From an economic perspective, the sensitivity of an early nonpregnancy test (ie, correct identification of pregnant cows) is more important than the specificity (ie, correct identification of nonpregnant cows) based on an economic simulation.[1] Inaccurate diagnosis of nonpregnancy (ie, false negatives), however, increases the rate of iatrogenic pregnancy loss when prostaglandin $F_{2\alpha}$ ($PGF_{2\alpha}$) or one of its analogues is administered to synchronize estrus or ovulation to reduce the interval to the next artificial insemination (AI) service. The economic loss incurred because of pregnancy loss depends on many factors and has been estimated to range from \$46[2] to \$300.[3] Because a management intervention can only be implemented for nonpregnant cows, it is critical that a pregnancy test accurately identify nonpregnant cows to avoid iatrogenic pregnancy loss. Nonetheless, a high rate of false-positive results diminishes the usefulness and cost-effectiveness of an early pregnancy test by failing to present a management opportunity to return nonpregnant cows to AI service early after AI and potentially increasing the interval to the subsequent AI.

RETURN TO ESTRUS AS A DIAGNOSTIC INDICATOR OF PREGNANCY STATUS

Accurate identification of cows returning to estrus from 18 to 32 days after AI is the easiest and least costly method for determining nonpregnancy early after insemination. This assumption, however, is being challenged by new research and long-recognized reproductive problems. First, estrous detection efficiency is estimated to be less than 50% on most dairy farms in the United States.[4] Only 51.5% of the eligible cows were detected in estrus and inseminated in a recent study in which detection of estrus was performed through continuous monitoring with activity tags after a previous insemination until pregnancy diagnosis 32 ±3 days after AI.[5] Second, estrous cycle duration varies widely with a high degree of variability among individual cows.[6] Finally, the high rate of pregnancy loss in dairy cows can increase the interval from insemination to return to estrus for cows that establish pregnancy early then undergo pregnancy loss later during gestation.[7]

PREGNANCY LOSS IN LACTATING DAIRY COWS

Pregnancy loss contributes to reproductive inefficiency because fertility assessed at any point during pregnancy is a function of both conception rate and pregnancy loss.[8] Pregnancy loss can be monitored using a variety of methods, including measurement of milk progesterone concentration or pregnancy-specific proteins, transrectal ultrasonography, and transrectal palpation. Since the widespread application of transrectal ultrasonography for reproductive research in cattle,[9] many studies have reported rates of pregnancy loss during early gestation under field conditions. In a summary of 14 studies,[10] pregnancy loss from 27 to 31 and 38 to 50 days of gestation averaged 13% based on transrectal ultrasonography. Vasconcelos and colleagues[11] characterized pregnancy loss at various stages of gestation using transrectal ultrasonography and reported pregnancy losses of 11% from 28 to 42 days, 6% from 42 to 56 days, and 2% from 56 to 98 days after AI (**Fig. 1**), supporting that the rate of loss is greater early during gestation and then decreases as gestation proceeds.

It has long been accepted that pregnancy status should be determined in dairy cows as soon as possible after insemination but without having the diagnosis confounded by subsequent pregnancy loss.[12,13] Pregnancy loss diminishes the benefit of early pregnancy diagnosis. Because of the high rate of pregnancy loss that occurs around the gestational period that most direct and indirect pregnancy tests are performed, the magnitude of pregnancy loss observed is greater the earlier after breeding that a positive diagnosis is made. Thus, the earlier that pregnancy is diagnosed after insemination, the fewer nonpregnant cows are identified to which a management strategy can be implemented to reinseminate them. If left unidentified, cows diagnosed pregnant early after insemination that subsequently undergo pregnancy loss decreases reproductive efficiency by extending the interval from calving to the insemination that results in a full-term pregnancy.

To compensate for pregnancy loss, cows diagnosed pregnant early after insemination must undergo one or more subsequent pregnancy examinations to identify and reinseminate cows that experience pregnancy loss. Most dairy farms conduct an early nonpregnancy diagnosis around 28 to 35 days after AI and then reconfirm pregnancies

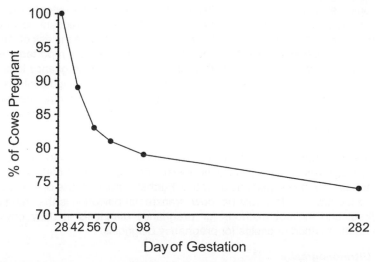

Fig. 1. Pregnancy loss in lactating Holstein cows assessed using transrectal ultrasonography from 28 days after AI to calving. (*Adapted from* Vasconcelos JLM, Silcox RW, Lacerda JA, et al. Pregnancy rate, pregnancy loss, and response to heat stress after AI at two different times from ovulation in dairy cows [abstract]. Biol Reprod 1997;56(Suppl 1):140; with permission.)

for cows diagnosed pregnant around 4 to 6 weeks later and around dry off to identify cows that have lost pregnancies. For many herds, particularly those with low estrus detection efficiency, pregnancy reconfirmation is critical to reinseminate cows that undergo pregnancy loss. Problems caused by pregnancy loss apply to all currently available methods for assessing pregnancy status early after breeding and may make pregnancy testing before 25 days after insemination impractical unless pregnancy diagnoses can be made continually and cost-effective on a daily basis or at each milking until the rate of pregnancy loss decreases or until the underlying causes of pregnancy loss are understood and mitigated.

DIRECT METHODS FOR PREGNANCY DIAGNOSIS

By definition, direct methods for early pregnancy diagnosis involve direct detection of the tissues and/or associated fluids of the conceptus either manually or via electronic instrumentation. Currently used direct methods for diagnosis of pregnancy include transrectal palpation and B-mode ultrasonography. Technical expertise, operator proficiency, and the stage after insemination that the technique is performed can affect the specificity and sensitivity of the test; however, experienced bovine practitioners can achieve high sensitivity and specificity with either method.

Transrectal Palpation

Transrectal palpation of the uterus for pregnancy diagnosis in cattle was first described in the 1800s[14] and is the oldest and most widely used direct method for early pregnancy diagnosis in dairy cows. Transrectal palpation of the amniotic vesicle as an aid in determining pregnancy status in dairy cows was described by Wisnicky and Cassida,[15] whereas slipping of the chorioallantoic membranes between the thumb and forefinger beginning on about 30 days in gestation was described by Zemjanis.[16]

Because pregnancy in cows can be intentionally terminated by manual rupture of the amnionic vesicle,[17,18] several studies have investigated the extent of iatrogenic pregnancy loss induced by transrectal palpation. Examining pregnant cows early in gestation by transrectal palpation has been reported to increase the risk of iatrogenic pregnancy loss in some studies,[19–23] whereas other studies have reported that cows submitted for transrectal palpation had a decreased risk for pregnancy loss or that palpation had no effect on subsequent pregnancy loss.[12,24] Although controversy still exists regarding the extent of iatrogenic pregnancy loss induced by transrectal palpation, other factors have a greater influence on calving rates than pregnancy examination using transrectal palpation.[25]

Because of its widespread use and the number of bovine practitioners trained to perform the procedure, transrectal palpation will likely remain a popular method for pregnancy diagnosis in dairy cows until newer direct or indirect methods for pregnancy diagnosis are developed and adopted. Furthermore, because of its widespread use, high accuracy, and low cost per cow, transrectal palpation is the standard that newer direct and indirect methods for pregnancy diagnosis in dairy cows must displace as the method of choice for pregnancy diagnosis.

B-Mode Ultrasonography

Applications of and detailed methods for performing transrectal ultrasonography for reproductive research have been extensively reviewed and described elsewhere.[8,9,26] Although early pregnancy diagnosis is among the most practical application for reproductive management using transrectal ultrasonography, additional information gathered using the technology that may be useful for reproductive management include evaluation of ovarian structures, identification of cows carrying twin fetuses, and determination of fetal sex.[8] Recently, changes in endometrial thickness using transrectal ultrasonography near the time of AI were reported to be a good indicator of ovulation failure and pregnancy success.[27] Transrectal ultrasonography has not been implicated as a direct cause of pregnancy loss in cows,[28,29] and ultrasound is a less invasive technique for early pregnancy diagnosis than is transrectal palpation.[21,22]

As a pregnancy diagnosis method, transrectal ultrasonography is accurate and rapid; the outcome of the test is known immediately at the time the test is conducted. Transrectal ultrasonography has begun to displace transrectal palpation as the direct method of choice by veterinarians for pregnancy diagnosis.[30] Because many experienced bovine practitioners can accurately diagnose pregnancy as early as 35 days after insemination using transrectal palpation, pregnancy examination using transrectal ultrasonography 28 to 34 days after insemination only reduces the interval from insemination to pregnancy diagnosis by a few days. Although ultrasound conducted at 45 or more days after breeding did not increase the accuracy of pregnancy diagnosis for an experienced palpator, it may improve diagnostic accuracy of a less experienced one.[31] The rate of pregnancy loss and the efficacy of strategies to reinseminate cows at various stages after breeding also play a role in determining the advantages and disadvantages on the timing of pregnancy diagnosis and resynchronization.[32]

Another potential benefit of transrectal ultrasonography over transrectal palpation is the opportunity to more accurately determine the ovarian status of cows at a nonpregnancy diagnosis facilitating the assignment of cows to different treatment alternatives. For example, use of an Ovsynch protocol for resynchronization of cows identified not pregnant 32 days after AI resulted in greater conception rates when cows were identified with a corpus luteum (CL) compared with cows without a CL at the first gonadotropin-releasing hormone (GnRH) treatment of the protocol.[33,34] Treatment of cows without a CL at the first GnRH treatment of an Ovsynch protocol with exogenous progesterone (ie, a intravaginal progesterone insert) increased fertility at first as well as resynch timed AI in lactating dairy cows.[35,36] Treatment of cows with a CL of 20 mm or greater at nonpregnancy diagnosis with a $PGF_{2\alpha}$ injection increased the overall proportion of cows inseminated after a detected estrus for second and subsequent AI services.[5] Based on these data, many veterinarians now use the presence or absence of a CL at a nonpregnancy diagnosis to improve outcomes to timed AI protocols used to resynchronize nonpregnant cows or to increase the proportion of cows inseminated in estrus after a previous insemination.

Problems with Early Pregnancy Diagnosis Using Transrectal Ultrasonography

Early studies in which transrectal ultrasonography was used to assess embryonic development in vivo reported that a fetal heartbeat could be visualized at around 21 days in gestation under controlled experimental conditions and using a high-quality scanner and transducer.[37] Several studies reported that pregnancy diagnosis can be rapidly and accurately diagnosed using ultrasound as early as 26 days after AI.[38,39] A recent report evaluated using transrectal ultrasonography as early as 18 to 21 days after insemination in Irish Holstein Friesian dairy cows.[40] Because of these reports, many bovine practitioners focused on pushing the lower limit of early pregnancy diagnosis to conduct pregnancy diagnosis using transrectal ultrasonography. Use of transrectal ultrasonography before about 30 days after insemination under field conditions on a commercial dairy, however, can negatively affect the accuracy of pregnancy diagnosis outcomes.[41]

To determine the accuracy of early pregnancy diagnosis using transrectal ultrasonography, we conducted a field trial on a commercial dairy farm milking approximately 2000 cows.[41] Pregnancy status was determined 29 days after timed AI using transrectal ultrasonography (Easi-scan, BCF Technology Ltd, Rochester, MN) based on the following criteria: presence or absence of a CL; presence, absence, volume, and appearance of uterine fluid typical for a 29-day conceptus; presence or absence of an embryo with a heartbeat. Cows were classified as (1) not pregnant: presence or absence of a CL, absence of uterine fluid or insufficient uterine fluid, and absence of an embryo; (2) pregnant: CL present, normal uterine fluid, and no embryo; (3) pregnant embryo: CL present, normal uterine fluid, and at least one embryo visualized; and (4) questionable pregnant: CL present and one or more of the following: uterine fluid, insufficient uterine fluid, and either no embryo or a nonviable embryo. At 39 and 74 days after timed AI, pregnancy status was determined using transrectal palpation and pregnancy loss occurring between each pregnancy examination was calculated.

Results from this experiment are shown in **Table 1**. Overall, 802 cows were classified as not pregnant 29 days after timed AI, whereas 799 cows were classified as not pregnant 39 days after timed AI resulting in a not-pregnant misdiagnosis rate of 0.5% (4 of 802) for transrectal ultrasonography 29 days after timed AI. At 29 days after timed AI, 1116 cows were classified as either pregnant with an embryo visualized (68%), pregnant based on uterine fluid alone (29%), or questionable pregnant (3%). Among questionable pregnant cows, 69% were classified as not pregnant 39 days after timed AI and an additional 46% were classified as not pregnant 74 days after timed AI. For cows classified pregnant 29 days after timed AI, more ($P<0.01$) cows diagnosed based on uterine fluid only than fluid and the presence of an embryo were classified as not pregnant using transrectal palpation 39 days after timed AI. Similarly, more ($P<0.01$) cows diagnosed pregnant based on uterine fluid alone than cows diagnosed pregnant based on visualization of an embryo with a heartbeat were classified as not pregnant

Table 1
Pregnancy loss by pregnancy classification for lactating Holstein cows diagnosed pregnant using ultrasonography 29 days after timed AI

	Pregnancy Classification[b]		
	Pregnant	Uterine Fluid	Questionable
Item		% (n/n)	
29 d after timed AI	68 (758 of 1116)	29 (322 of 1116)	3 (36 of 1116)
Pregnancy loss			
29–39 d	4[a] (30 of 758)	18[a] (57 of 322)	69[a] (25 of 36)
39–74 d	5[a] (39 of 728)	12[a] (32 of 265)	46[a] (5 of 11)
Total loss	9[a] (69 of 758)	28[a] (89 of 322)	83[a] (30 of 36)

[a] Within a row, proportions with different superscripts differ ($P<.001$).
[b] Lactating Holstein cows diagnosed pregnant were classified based on the following criteria using transrectal ultrasonography: pregnant: visualization of a CL ipsilateral to the gravid uterine horn, visualization of an amount of nonechogenic uterine fluid in accordance to stage of pregnancy, and visualization of an embryo with a heartbeat; uterine fluid: visualization of a CL ipsilateral to the gravid uterine horn, visualization of an amount of nonechogenic uterine fluid in accordance to stage of pregnancy but without visualization of the embryo; questionable: visualization of a CL ipsilateral to the gravid uterine horn with insufficient uterine fluid for the stage of pregnancy.
Adapted from Giordano JO, Fricke PM. Accuracy of pregnancy diagnosis outcomes using transrectal ultrasonography 29 days after artificial insemination in lactating dairy cows. J Dairy Sci 2012;95(Suppl 2):75; with permission.

using transrectal palpation 74 days after timed AI. From the initial pregnancy examination at 29 days to the last examination 74 days after timed AI, more ($P<0.01$) cows diagnosed pregnant based on uterine fluid alone than cows diagnosed pregnant based on visualization of an embryo with a heartbeat were classified as not pregnant using transrectal palpation 74 days after timed AI. Cows classified pregnant based on uterine fluid alone 29 days after timed AI were 3.8 (95% confidence interval = 2.7–5.4) times more likely to be classified as not pregnant 74 days after timed AI than cows diagnosed pregnant based on visualization of an embryo with a heartbeat.

Based on these data, the authors concluded that the accuracy of pregnancy outcomes using transrectal ultrasonography increase dramatically when an embryo with a heartbeat is visualized compared with outcomes based only on the presence of a CL and the volume of uterine fluid in the absence of a visualized embryo with a heartbeat. The presence of a large proportion of cows with a CL and fluid was visualized in the absence of an embryo with a heartbeat is likely due to a high degree of early pregnancy loss in dairy cows. In 2 experiments, 35% to 44% of dairy cows diagnosed not pregnant 32 days after timed AI had extended luteal phases.[7,42] Based on the authors' results, early pregnancy diagnosis should not be conducted earlier than an embryo with a heartbeat can be rapidly and reliably detected in pregnant cows under on-farm conditions using transrectal ultrasonography (~30 days after AI) to reduce the negative impact of false-positive results.

INDIRECT METHODS FOR PREGNANCY DIAGNOSIS IN DAIRY COWS

Indirect methods for early pregnancy diagnosis use qualitative or quantitative measures of hormones or conceptus-specific substances in maternal body fluids as indirect indicators of the presence of a viable pregnancy. Commercially available indirect methods for pregnancy diagnosis in dairy cows include milk progesterone tests and tests for pregnancy-associated glycoproteins (PAGs) in blood or milk.

Progesterone

Progesterone is the most biologically active progestagen in cattle and is primarily produced and secreted by the corpus luteum during the estrous cycle and the placenta during pregnancy. Quantification of progesterone in blood or milk can be achieved in a laboratory using radioimmunoassay (RIA) or enzyme-linked immunosorbent assay (ELISA) methods. The biology of early pregnancy and maintenance of the CL results in distinct progesterone profiles for pregnant compared with nonpregnant cows. Lactating dairy cows were synchronized for first timed AI, and resulting progesterone profiles based on thrice weekly (Monday, Wednesday, Friday) blood sampling are shown in **Fig. 2**. The upper panel of **Fig. 2** indicates a cow that failed to become pregnant and had a normal luteal phase followed by a subsequent estrous cycle. By contrast, the middle panel of **Fig. 2** indicates a cow that maintained pregnancy. The lower panel of **Fig. 2** is representative of cows that fail to maintain a pregnancy and had an extended luteal phase. Extended luteal phases are common in dairy cows after AI. In one experiment, 35% of dairy cows diagnosed not pregnant 32 days after timed AI had extended luteal phases[42]; in another experiment, the proportion of cows with extended luteal phases was 44%.[7] Unfortunately, sequential sampling of milk or blood for determination of progesterone using RIA or ELISA methods is not practical or cost-effective for use on commercial dairy farms. Future technologies to monitor milk progesterone profiles of individual cows on a daily or even a weekly basis could revolutionize reproductive management strategies for dairy cows.

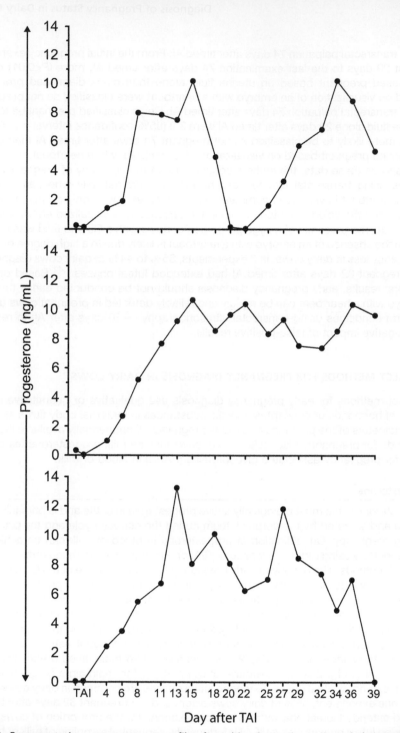

Fig. 2. Representative progesterone profiles from blood samples collected thrice weekly (Monday, Wednesday, Friday) from Holstein dairy cows after synchronization of ovulation and timed AI. Upper panel: a cow that failed to become pregnant after timed AI and had a normal luteal phase; middle panel: a cow that became pregnant after timed AI; lower panel: a cow that failed to become pregnant after timed AI and had an extended luteal phase.

Rapid on-farm qualitative tests for assessing progesterone levels in milk were commercialized for pregnancy diagnosis in dairy cows in the 1980s,[43] and a few remain commercially available today. Manufacturers recommended these tests be conducted 18 to 24 days after insemination to determine pregnancy status. Based on the progesterone profiles in **Fig. 2**, cows with low progesterone 18 to 24 days after AI would be classified as not pregnant, whereas cows with high progesterone 18 to 24 days after AI would be classified as pregnant. Although not-pregnant outcomes are highly accurate for identifying cows that truly are not pregnant, the accuracy of high progesterone 18 to 24 days after AI for accurately diagnosing pregnant cows is poor. This poor accuracy is due to the biology associated with pregnancy loss that confounds early pregnancy diagnosis using transrectal ultrasonography discussed previously. Most of these extended luteal phases may be explained by cows that establish a pregnancy early by signaling maternal recognition of pregnancy and maintenance of the CL past the normal time of luteal regression but then subsequently undergo pregnancy loss.[7] Thus, although future technologies may allow for on-farm sampling of milk progesterone, the use of cow-side milk progesterone tests conducted 18 to 24 days after insemination should focus on identifying not-pregnant cows rather than pregnant cows.

Pregnancy-Associated Proteins

Proteins produced and secreted by the placenta early during pregnancy are obvious candidates for development of an early pregnancy test; however, proteins produced by the placenta vary widely among eutherotic mammals. For example, only the higher primates produce a chorionic gonadotropin homologous to the human protein (human chorionic gonadotropin) required for luteal support early during pregnancy, whereas only ruminant ungulates are known to produce type I interferon as an antiluteolytic hormone.[44] Because cattle do not produce a chorionic gonadotropin, research has focused on discovery and characterization of pregnancy-specific proteins suitable for determining pregnancy status in cattle early after insemination. Some pregnancy-associated factors, such as the early conception factor, have not proven to be accurate in dairy cows.[45] It is now possible to detect a viable conceptus between 15 to 22 days after AI by measuring the expression of interferon-stimulated genes in circulating white blood cells[46–48]; however, this method has not yet been commercialized. The most recent advance in this area has been made in the commercialization of tests for PAGs.

Pregnancy-Associated Glycoproteins

Bovine PAGs were discovered through attempts to develop indirect early pregnancy tests in dairy cows.[44] In 1982, two proteins, pregnancy-specific protein (PSP) A and B, were isolated from bovine fetal membrane extracts.[49] Development of a specific RIA for PSPB[50] allowed for quantification of PSPB in maternal serum as an indirect method for pregnancy diagnosis and pregnancy loss in dairy cows.[51,52] Molecular cloning and sequencing studies revealed that PAGs belong to a large family of inactive aspartic proteinases expressed by the placenta of domestic ruminants, including cows, ewes, and goats.[53]

In cattle, the PAG gene family comprises at least 22 transcribed genes as well as some variants.[54] Bovine PAGs have been immunologically localized to trophoblast binucleate cells present in fetal cotyledonary villi and to a lesser extent to caruncular epithelium.[55] Migration of binucleate cells from the trophectoderm to the uterine epithelium allows for exocytosis of granules containing PAG into the maternal circulation.[56] Because cellular products of binucleate cells are released into maternal circulation, the ideal antigen for an indirect early pregnancy test in dairy cows would be a PAG expressed in binucleate cells around the time of implantation.[57] Mean PAG concentrations in cattle increase from 15 to 35 days in gestation[42]; however, variation in plasma PAG levels among cows precludes PAG testing as a reliable indicator of pregnancy until about 26 to 30 days after AI.[58,59] Several experiments have evaluated the use of commercial PAG tests to determine pregnancy status in dairy cows and heifers (**Table 2**). The sensitivity, specificity, positive predictive value (PPV), negative predictive value (NPV), and accuracy obtained using PAG tests are summarized based on several experiments[58,60–66] in **Table 2**.

Few studies have compared factors associated with PAG levels in blood and milk of dairy cows early in gestation and the impact these factors may have on the accuracy of pregnancy diagnosis. The authors recently conducted an experiment to determine the factors affecting PAG levels in blood and milk of dairy cows during early gestation.[66] Lactating Holstein cows (n = 141) were synchronized to receive their first timed artificial AI. Blood and milk samples were collected 25 and 32 days after timed AI (TAI), and pregnancy status was determined 32 days after TAI using transrectal ultrasonography. Cows diagnosed pregnant with singletons (n = 48) continued the experiment in which blood and milk samples were collected, and pregnancy status was assessed weekly using transrectal ultrasonography from 39 to 102 days after TAI. Plasma and milk samples were assayed for PAG levels using commercial ELISA kits.

Table 2
Sensitivity, specificity, PPV, NPV, and accuracy for RIA and ELISA PAG test results

Reference	Days After AI	Test	Sensitivity[a]	Specificity[b]	PPV[c]	NPV[d]	Accuracy[e]
Zoli et al,[58] 1992	22–30	RIA (blood PAG)	98.8	87.5	93.0	97.9	94.5
Szenci et al,[60] 1998	26–58	RIA (PSPB)	75–100	85–92	81–91	80–100	80–96
		RIA (blood PAG)	81–100	57–71	62–74	78–100	69–84
Silva et al,[61] 2007	27	ELISA (blood PAG)	94–96	92–97	90–98	97–98	94–96
Romano & Larson,[62] 2010	28–35	ELISA (PSPB)	94–97	94–96	92–95	95–98	95–96
Piechotta et al,[63] 2011	26–58	ELISA (PSPB)	98.0	97.1	99.3	91.9	97.8
		ELISA (blood PAG)	97.8	91.2	97.8	91.2	96.4
Sinedino et al,[64] 2014	28	ELISA (blood PAG)	95	89	90	95	92
Lawson et al,[65] 2014	30–95	ELISA (milk PAG)	98–100	98–100	99–100	83–100	98–100
Ricci et al,[66] 2015	32	ELISA (blood PAG)	100	87	84	100	92
		ELISA (milk PAG)	98	83	79	99	89

Abbreviations: NPV, negative predictive value; PAG, pregnancy-associated glycoprotein; PPV, positive predictive value; PSPB, pregnancy specific protein B.
[a] Proportion of serum samples from pregnant cows with a positive PAG test result.
[b] Proportion of serum samples from nonpregnant cows with a negative PAG test result.
[c] Probability that a positive PAG test result is from a pregnant cow.
[d] Probability that a negative PAG test result is from a nonpregnant cow.
[e] Probability of correctly identifying pregnancy status.

To evaluate pregnancy outcomes from the plasma and milk PAG tests in cows of unknown pregnancy status, 2 by 2 contingency tables were constructed to calculate sensitivity, specificity, PPV, NPV, and accuracy of the pregnancy outcomes for the plasma and milk PAG tests 32 days after timed AI; these outcomes were compared with those based on transrectal ultrasonography 32 days after timed AI (**Table 3**). Sensitivity for both the plasma and milk PAG tests in the present experiment was high (100% and 98%, respectively) compared with specificity (87% and 83%, respectively). As a result, the NPV for the plasma and milk PAG tests in the present experiment was high (100% and 99%, respectively) compared with the PPV of both tests (84% and 79%, respectively). The overall accuracy of the plasma and milk PAG tests 32 days after timed AI was 92% and 89%, respectively. Results from this sensitivity analysis support that the accuracy of using plasma or milk PAG levels as an indicator of pregnancy status in dairy cows 32 days after AI is high, and the authors' results agree with others who have conducted similar analyses from 27 to 39 days in gestation when PAG levels in both plasma and milk are at early peak levels.[61,64,65]

The incidence of pregnancy loss in the present study for cows diagnosed with singleton pregnancies 32 days after TAI during the experiment was 13% (7 of 55), which agrees with the 13% loss reported to occur from 27 to 31 and 38 to 50 days of gestation based on transrectal ultrasonography in a summary of 14 studies.[10] For the plasma PAG ELISA, all but one cow that underwent pregnancy loss tested positive, whereas all cows undergoing pregnancy loss tested positive at one or more time points for the milk PAG test. Similarly, 5 of 7 cows tested recheck based on the plasma PAG test before the loss occurred compared with 3 of 7 cows based on the milk PAG test. Thus, PAG levels detected by these ELISA tests in the present study have a half-life in maternal circulation resulting in a 7- to 14-day delay in identification of cows undergoing pregnancy loss based on plasma or milk PAG levels compared with transrectal ultrasonography.

Profiles of PAG in plasma and milk of cows that maintained pregnancy from 25 to 102 days in gestation are shown in **Fig. 3**. Compared with transrectal ultrasonography, accuracy was 92% for the plasma PAG test and 89% for the milk PAG test 32 days after timed AI. Factors associated with PAG levels in dairy cows included stage of gestation, parity, pregnancy loss, and milk production. Based on plasma and milk PAG profiles, the optimal time to conduct a first pregnancy diagnosis is around 32 days after AI coinciding with an early peak in PAG levels. The authors concluded that because of the

Table 3
Sensitivity, specificity, PPV, NPV, and accuracy of plasma and milk PAG ELISA tests for determination of pregnancy status 32 days after AI

PAG ELISA	PPV[a] % (No./No.)	NPV[b] % (No./No.)	Sensitivity[c] % (No./No.)	Specificity[d] % (No./No.)	Accuracy[e] % (No./No.)
Plasma	84 (57 of 68)	100 (73 of 73)	100 (57 of 57)	87 (73 of 84)	92 (130 of 141)
Milk	79 (52 of 66)	99 (68 of 69)	98 (52 of 53)	83 (68 of 82)	89 (120 of 135)

[a] Proportion of cows diagnosed pregnant using the PAG ELISA that truly were pregnant.
[b] Proportion of cows diagnosed as not pregnant using the PAG ELISA that truly were not pregnant.
[c] Proportion of pregnant cows with a positive PAG ELISA outcome.
[d] Proportion of not-pregnant cows with a negative PAG ELISA outcome.
[e] Proportion of pregnancy status outcomes, pregnant and not pregnant, that were correctly classified by the PAG ELISA.
Adapted from Ricci A, Carvalho PD, Amundson MC, et al. Factors associated with pregnancy-associated glycoprotein (PAG) levels in plasma and milk of Holstein cows during early pregnancy and their effect on the accuracy of pregnancy diagnosis. J Dairy Sci 2015;98:2502–14; with permission.

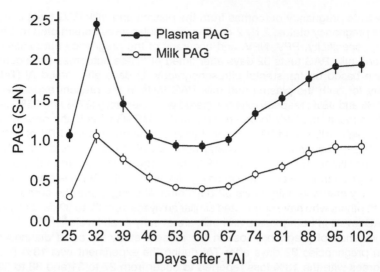

Fig. 3. Plasma and milk PAG profiles for Holstein dairy cows (n = 48) that maintained pregnancy from 25 to 102 days after AI. ELISA outcomes were calculated from the optical density (OD) of the sample (corrected by subtraction of the reference wavelength OD of the sample [S] minus the OD of the negative control [N] at 450 nm with both values corrected by subtraction of the reference wavelength OD of the negative control), which resulted in an S-N value. Plasma and milk PAG levels were affected by week after AI (*P*<.01). (*Adapted from* Ricci A, Carvalho PD, Amundson MC, et al. Factors associated with pregnancy-associated glycoprotein (PAG) levels in plasma and milk of Holstein cows during early pregnancy and their effect on the accuracy of pregnancy diagnosis. J Dairy Sci 2015;98:2502–14; with permission.)

occurrence of pregnancy loss, all pregnant cows should be retested 74 days after AI or later when plasma and milk PAG levels in pregnant cows have rebounded from their nadir.

FUTURE TECHNOLOGIES FOR PREGNANCY DIAGNOSIS

A novel approach to the problem of early pregnancy diagnosis in dairy cows would be to monitor a pregnancy-specific substance or hormone secreted in milk in sufficient quantities to be detected by an in-line milk-sensing device during normal milking periods on a dairy. Obviously, this pregnancy-specific substance must first be discovered or a known marker must be used and the in-line milk sampling technology developed to accurately detect and monitor this substance. If sensitive and specific, such a system would have a minimal marginal cost per test once the initial capital outlay was made to install the equipment on the dairy. By using such a system, a pregnancy diagnosis would be conducted during each milking period for all lactating cows on a dairy so that nonpregnancy, pregnancy, and pregnancy loss could be continually monitored and tracked on a daily basis. Integration of this information into a computerized dairy management software system would allow dairy managers to review the pregnancy status of individual cows in the herd on a daily or weekly basis so that reproductive management strategies could be implemented to establish, maintain, or attempt to reinitiate a pregnancy. Finally, such a system would achieve the heretofore-unrealized characteristic of conducting the pregnancy test without having to handle the cow to administer the test. Limitations imposed by pregnancy loss during early gestation will not be overcome until such a system is developed.

SUMMARY

Although coupling a nonpregnancy diagnosis with a management strategy to quickly reinitiate AI may improve reproductive efficiency by decreasing the interval between AI services, early pregnancy loss limits the accuracy of many direct and indirect methods for early pregnancy diagnosis currently under development. These limitations make the benefits of many currently available methods for early pregnancy diagnosis questionable and require that all cows diagnosed pregnant early after insemination be scheduled for pregnancy reconfirmations at later times during gestation to identify cows experiencing pregnancy loss. Although much research and development efforts are being made toward development of an indirect pregnancy test for dairy cows, it remains to be seen whether these indirect tests will replace transrectal palpation or transrectal ultrasonography as the primary method used for pregnancy diagnosis in dairy cows or whether veterinarians will combine these methods in a reproductive management program. Future technologies for pregnancy diagnosis in dairy cows may someday overcome current limitations of direct and indirect methods for pregnancy diagnosis, thereby improving reproductive performance.

REFERENCES

1. Giordano JO, Fricke PM, Cabrera VE. Economics of resynchronization strategies including chemical tests to identify nonpregnant cows. J Dairy Sci 2013;96: 949–61.
2. Ferguson JD, Galligan DT. The value of pregnancy diagnosis—a revisit to an old art. Annual Conference Symposium. Society of Theriogenology. Montgomery, AL; Milwaukee, WI. August 9–13, 2011.
3. Galligan DT, Ferguson J, Munson R, et al. Economic concepts regarding early pregnancy testing. In: Proceedings of the American Association of Bovine Practitioners. Omaha, NE; Auburn, AL. 2009. p. 48–53.
4. Senger PL. The estrus detection problem: new concepts, technologies, and possibilities. J Dairy Sci 1994;77:2745–53.
5. Giordano JO, Stangaferro ML, Wijma R, et al. Reproductive performance of dairy cows managed with a program aimed at increasing insemination of cows in estrus based on increased physical activity and fertility of timed artificial inseminations. J Dairy Sci 2015;98:2488–501.
6. Remnant JG, Green MJ, Huxley JN, et al. Variation in the interservice intervals of dairy cows in the United Kingdom. J Dairy Sci 2015;98:889–97.
7. Ricci A, Carvalho PD, Amundson MC, et al. Characterization of luteal dynamics in lactating dairy cows for 32 days after synchronization of ovulation and timed artificial insemination. J Dairy Sci 2014;97(Suppl 1):693.
8. Fricke PM. Scanning the future – ultrasonography as a reproductive management tool for dairy cattle. J Dairy Sci 2002;85:1918–26.
9. Griffin PG, Ginther OJ. Research applications of ultrasonic imaging in reproductive biology. J Anim Sci 1992;70:953–72.
10. Santos JEP, Thatcher WW, Chebel RC, et al. The effect of embryonic death rates in cattle on the efficacy of estrus synchronization programs. Anim Reprod Sci 2004;82–83:513–35.
11. Vasconcelos JLM, Silcox RW, Lacerda JA, et al. Pregnancy rate, pregnancy loss, and response to heat stress after AI at two different times from ovulation in dairy cows [abstract]. Biol Reprod 1997;56(Suppl 1):140.
12. Studer E. Early pregnancy diagnosis and fetal death. Vet Med Small Anim Clin 1969;64:613–7.

13. Melrose DR. The need for, and possible methods of application of, hormone assay techniques for improving reproductive efficiency. Br Vet J 1979;135:453–9.

14. Cowie TA. Pregnancy diagnosis tests: a review. Commonwealth agricultural bureaux joint publication No. 13, Oxford, UK; 1948. p. 11–7.

15. Wisnicky W, Cassida LE. A manual method for diagnosis of pregnancy in cattle. J Am Vet Med Assoc 1948;113:451.

16. Zemjanis R. Diagnostic and therapeutic techniques in animal reproduction. 2nd edition. Baltimore (MD): Williams and Wilkins; 1970. p. 29–45.

17. Ball L, Carroll EJ. Induction of fetal death in cattle by manual rupture of the amniotic vesicle. J Am Vet Med Assoc 1963;142:373–4.

18. López-Gatius F. The effect on pregnancy rate of progesterone administration after manual reduction of twin embryos in dairy cattle. J Vet Med A Physiol Pathol Clin Med 2005;52:199–201.

19. Abbitt BL, Ball G, Kitto P, et al. Effect of three methods of palpation for pregnancy diagnosis per rectum on embryonic and fetal attrition in cows. J Am Vet Med Assoc 1978;173:973–7.

20. Franco OJ, Drost M, Thatcher MJ, et al. Fetal survival in the cow after pregnancy diagnosis by palpation per rectum. Theriogenology 1987;27:631–44.

21. Paisley LG, Mickelsen WD, Frost OL. A survey of the incidence of prenatal mortality in cattle following pregnancy diagnosis by rectal palpation. Theriogenology 1978;9:481–9.

22. Vaillancourt D, Vierschwal CJ, Ogwu D, et al. Correlation between pregnancy diagnosis by membrane slip and embryonic mortality. J Am Vet Med Assoc 1979;175:466–8.

23. White ME, LaFaunce N, Mohammed HO. Calving outcomes for cows diagnosed pregnant or nonpregnant by per rectum examination at various intervals after insemination. Can Vet J 1989;30:867–70.

24. Thurmond MC, Picanso JP. Fetal loss associated with palpation per rectum to diagnose pregnancy in cows. J Am Vet Med Assoc 1993;203:432–5.

25. Thompson JA, Marsh WE, Calvin JA, et al. Pregnancy attrition associated with pregnancy testing by rectal palpation. J Dairy Sci 1994;77:3382–7.

26. Ginther OJ. Ultrasonic imaging and animal reproduction: cattle. Book 3. Cross Plains (WI): Equiservices Publishing; 1998.

27. Souza AH, Silva EPB, Cunha AP, et al. Ultrasonographic evaluation of endometrial thickness near timed AI as a predictor of fertility in high-producing dairy cows. Theriogenology 2011;75:722–33.

28. Ball PJH, Logue DDN. Ultrasound diagnosis of pregnancy in cattle. Vet Rec 1994; 134:532.

29. Baxter SJ, Ward WR. Incidence of fetal loss in dairy cattle after pregnancy diagnosis using an ultrasound scanner. Vet Rec 1997;140:287–8.

30. Caraviello DZ, Weigel KA, Fricke PM, et al. Survey of management practices on reproductive performance of dairy cattle on large US commercial farms. J Dairy Sci 2006;89(12):4723–35.

31. Galland JC, Offenbach LA, Spire MF. Measuring the time needed to confirm fetal age in beef heifers using ultrasonographic examination. Vet Med 1994;89:795–804.

32. Fricke PM, Caraviello DZ, Weigel KA, et al. Fertility of dairy cows after resynchronization of ovulation at three intervals after first timed insemination. J Dairy Sci 2003;86:3941–50.

33. Giordano JO, Wiltbank MC, Guenther JN, et al. Increased fertility in lactating dairy cows resynchronized with Double-Ovsynch compared with Ovsynch initiated 32 d after timed artificial insemination. J Dairy Sci 2012;95:639–53.

34. Lopes G Jr, Giordano JO, Valenza A, et al. Effect of timing of initiation of resynchronization and presynchronization with gonadotropin-releasing hormone on fertility of resynchronized inseminations in lactating dairy cows. J Dairy Sci 2013;96:3788–98.
35. Chebel RC, Al-Hassan MJ, Fricke PM, et al. Supplementation of progesterone via controlled internal drug release inserts during ovulation synchronization protocols in lactating dairy cows. J Dairy Sci 2010;93:922–31.
36. Bilby TR, Brune RGS, Lager KJ, et al. Supplemental progesterone and timing of resynchronization on pregnancy outcomes in lactating dairy cows. J Dairy Sci 2013;96:7032–42.
37. Curran S, Pierson RA, Ginther OJ. Ultrasonographic appearance of the bovine conceptus from days 20 through 60. J Am Vet Med Assoc 1986;189:1295–302.
38. Pieterse MC, Szenci O, Willemse AH, et al. Early pregnancy diagnosis in cattle by means of linear-array real-time ultrasound scanning of the uterus and a qualitative and quantitative milk progesterone test. Theriogenology 1990;33:697–707.
39. Nation DP, Malmo J, Davis GM, et al. Accuracy of bovine pregnancy detection using transrectal ultrasonography at 28 to 35 days after insemination. Aust Vet J 2003;81:63–5.
40. Scully S, Butler ST, Kelly AK, et al. Early pregnancy diagnosis on days 18 to 21 postinsemination using high-resolution imaging in lactating dairy cows. J Dairy Sci 2014;97:3542–57.
41. Giordano JO, Fricke PM. Accuracy of pregnancy diagnosis outcomes using transrectal ultrasonography 29 days after artificial insemination in lactating dairy cows. J Dairy Sci 2012;95(Suppl 2):75.
42. Giordano JO, Guenther JN, Lopes G Jr, et al. Changes in serum pregnancy-associated glycoprotein, pregnancy-specific protein B, and progesterone concentrations before and after induction of pregnancy loss in lactating dairy cows. J Dairy Sci 2012;95:683–97.
43. Nebel RL. On-farm milk progesterone tests. J Dairy Sci 1988;71:1682–90.
44. Xie S, Green J, Bixby JB, et al. The diversity and evolutionary relationships of the pregnancy-associated glycoproteins, an aspartic proteinase subfamily consisting of many trophoblast-expressed genes. Proc Natl Acad Sci U S A 1997;94:12809–16.
45. Cordoba MC, Sartori R, Fricke PM. Assessment of a commercially available early conception factor (ECF) test for determining pregnancy status of dairy cattle. J Dairy Sci 2001;84:1884–9.
46. Stevenson JL, Dalton JC, Ott TL, et al. Correlation between reproductive status and steady-state messenger ribonucleic acid levels of the Myxovirus resistance gene, MX2, in peripheral blood leukocytes of dairy heifers. J Anim Sci 2007;85:2163–72.
47. Gifford CA, Racicot K, Clark DS, et al. Regulation of interferon-stimulated genes in peripheral blood leukocytes in pregnant and bred, nonpregnant dairy cows. J Dairy Sci 2008;90:274–80.
48. Green JC, Okamura CS, Poock SE, et al. Measurement of interferon-tau (IFN-τ) stimulated gene expression in blood leukocytes for pregnancy diagnosis within 18–20 d after insemination in dairy cattle. Anim Reprod Sci 2010;121:24–33.
49. Butler JE, Hamilton WC, Sasser RG, et al. Detection and partial characterization of two bovine pregnancy-specific proteins. Biol Reprod 1982;26:925–33.
50. Sasser RG, Ruder CA, Ivani KA, et al. Detection of pregnancy by radioimmunoassay of a novel pregnancy-specific protein in serum of cows and a profile of serum concentration during gestation. Biol Reprod 1986;35:936–42.
51. Humblot P, Camous S, Martal J, et al. Diagnosis of pregnancy by radioimmunoassay of a pregnancy-specific protein in the plasma of dairy cows. Theriogenology 1988;30:257–68.

52. Humblot P, Camous S, Martal J, et al. Pregnancy-specific protein B, progesterone concentrations and embryonic mortality during early pregnancy in dairy cows. J Reprod Fertil 1988;83:215–23.
53. Haugejorden G, Waage S, Dahl E, et al. Pregnancy associated glycoproteins (PAG) in postpartum cows, ewes, goats and their offspring. Theriogenology 2006;66:1976–84.
54. Prakash B, Telugu VL, Walker AM, et al. Characterization of the bovine pregnancy-associated glycoprotein gene family – analysis of gene sequences, regulatory regions within the promoter and expression of selected genes. BMC Genomics 2009;10:185–202.
55. Zoli AP, Demez P, Beckers JF, et al. Light and electron microscopic immunolocalization of bovine pregnancy-associated glycoprotein in the bovine placentome. Biol Reprod 1992;46:623–9.
56. Wooding FBP. Current topic: the synepitheliochorial placenta of ruminants: binucleate cell fusions and hormone production. Placenta 1992;13:101–13.
57. Green JA, Xie S, Quan X, et al. Pregnancy-associated bovine and ovine glycoproteins exhibit spatially and temporally distinct expression patterns during pregnancy. Biol Reprod 2000;62:1624–163131.
58. Zoli AP, Guilbault LA, Delahaut P, et al. Radioimmunoassay of a bovine pregnancy-associated glycoprotein in serum: its application for pregnancy diagnosis. Biol Reprod 1992;46:83–92.
59. Humblot P. Use of pregnancy specific proteins and progesterone assays to monitor pregnancy and determine the timing, frequencies and sources of embryonic mortality in ruminants. Theriogenology 2001;56:1417–33.
60. Szenci O, Beckers JF, Humblot P, et al. Comparison of ultrasonography, bovine pregnancy-specific protein B, and bovine pregnancy-associated glycoprotein 1 tests for pregnancy detection in dairy cows. Theriogenology 1998;50:77–88.
61. Silva E, Sterry RA, Kolb D, et al. Accuracy of a pregnancy-associated glycoprotein ELISA to determine pregnancy status of lactating dairy cows twenty-seven days after timed artificial insemination. J Dairy Sci 2007;90:4612–22.
62. Romano JE, Larson JE. Accuracy of pregnancy specific protein-B test for early pregnancy diagnosis in dairy cattle. Theriogenology 2010;74:932–9.
63. Piechotta M, Bollwein J, Friedrich M, et al. Comparison of commercial ELISA blood tests for early pregnancy detection in dairy cows. J Reprod Dev 2011;57:72–5.
64. Sinedino LDP, Lima FS, Bisinotto RS, et al. Effect of early or late resynchronization based on different methods of pregnancy diagnosis on reproductive performance of dairy cows. J Dairy Sci 2014;97:4932–41.
65. Lawson BC, Shahzad AH, Dolecheck KA, et al. A pregnancy detection assay using milk samples: evaluation and considerations. J Dairy Sci 2014;97:6316–25.
66. Ricci A, Carvalho PD, Amundson MC, et al. Factors associated with pregnancy-associated glycoprotein (PAG) levels in plasma and milk of Holstein cows during early pregnancy and their effect on the accuracy of pregnancy diagnosis. J Dairy Sci 2015;98:2502–14.

Practical Use of Ultrasound Scan in Small Ruminant Medicine and Surgery

Phil Scott, BVM&S, DVM&S, MPhil, DSHP, FHEA, FRCVS

KEYWORDS

- Ultrasound diagnosis • Sheep • Respiratory disease • Urolithiasis

KEY POINTS

- Ultrasound examination of particular organs takes no more than 5 minutes with the results available immediately.
- 5 MHz linear array scanners can be used for most organs except the heart and right kidney.
- Transthoracic ultrasonography is particularly useful for critical evaluation of lung and pleural pathologies.
- Transabdominal ultrasonographic examination can readily identify distended urinary bladder and advanced hydronephrosis.

 Videos of ultrasound examples accompany this article at http://www.vetfood. theclinics.com/

INTRODUCTION

Many veterinarians in food animal practice routinely use transrectal ultrasonographic examination for the early detection, and possibly sexing, of bovine embryos using 5-MHz linear array scanners. This equipment can also be used in adult sheep to provide diagnostic quality ultrasound images except for the kidney and heart; a 5- to 6.5-MHz sector scanner is often necessary in sheep less than 30 kg.

Transthoracic ultrasonography is particularly useful for critical evaluation of the lungs because auscultated adventitious sounds do not correlate well with lesion distribution in ovine pulmonary adenocarcinoma (OPA) and other respiratory tract pathologies.[1,2]

Transabdominal ultrasonography has been used successfully in commercial flocks for the past 30 years to determine fetal number and gestation length permitting more precise feeding and management during late gestation.[3–5] Ultrasonographic

The author has nothing to disclose.
Division of Veterinary Clinical Sciences, R(D)SVS, University of Edinburgh, Easter Bush, Roslin, Midlothian EH25 9RG, UK
E-mail address: Philip.R.Scott@ed.ac.uk

examination has yielded important clinical information regarding size of the abomasum to determine colostrum ingestion,[6] respiratory system,[7] joints,[8] bladder and kidney,[9] uterus,[10] peritoneum, and liver.[11] Ultrasound examination of vaginal prolapse has guided a more effective method for replacement when the urinary bladder is identified within the prolapsed tissues.[12] On-farm identification of distended bladder caused by urinary tract obstruction[9] enables immediate action without recourse to laboratory testing and further delays that adversely influence prognosis.

ULTRASONOGRAPHIC EXAMINATION—EQUIPMENT

A 5.0-MHz linear transducer connected to a real-time, B-mode ultrasound machine can be used for all ultrasonographic examinations in adult sheep except examination of the right kidney and heart, where a 5- to 6.5-MHz sector transducer is necessary to ensure good contact between the concave flank of the right sublumbar fossa and access to the fourth and fifth rib spaces, respectively. A field setting of 7 to 9 cm on the linear scanner is appropriate for most abdominal examinations; occasionally the 20-cm field depth afforded by certain 5.0- to 6.5-MHz sector scanners more accurately determines the extent of fluid accumulation and bladder diameter, but this does not significantly alter the clinical diagnosis. Transrectal examination of the bladder and rectum has been reported in both rams and ewes,[13,14] but this examination has not proved necessary to determine obstructive urolithiasis in clinical practice.

SITES FOR ULTRASONOGRAPHIC EXAMINATION
Chest

A 5- to 6.5-MHz sector transducer connected to a real-time, B-mode ultrasound machine is preferred for ultrasonographic examination of the chest. An initial field setting of 6 to 7 cm allows detailed examination of the pleurae and superficial lung parenchyma and can be subsequently increased to examine the full extent of any lesions (up to 12–16 cm). A 5-cm-wide strip of skin is quickly shaved from both sides of the thorax extending vertically from the point of the elbow; in many breeds the ventral margin of this area of skin has only fine hairs and no fleece. The skin is soaked with warm tap water then ultrasound gel liberally applied to the wet skin to ensure good contact. The transducer head is firmly held against the skin overlying the intercostal muscles of the fifth to seventh intercostal spaces, and the thorax examined in both longitudinal and transverse planes. The dorsal lung field is selected at the start of all ultrasound examinations in an attempt to visualize normal lung tissue, as this area is much less commonly affected in ovine respiratory disease.

Liver

The liver can be imaged from the seventh to eleventh intercostal spaces halfway down the right chest wall with the 5- to 6.5-MHz sector probe head pointed toward the contralateral shoulder.[11]

Bladder, Uterus, Vagina, and Ventral Abdomen

The absence of fleece in the ventral midline and inguinal area expedites preparation when examining the ventral and caudal abdomen in sheep. Ultrasonographic examination of the bladder and caudal abdomen are undertaken in the standing animal using either 5- to 6.5-MHz linear array or sector scanners. The caudal abdomen is examined for the bladder and gravid uterus. The right inguinal region is chosen because the left side of the abdomen is largely occupied by the rumen. The transducer head is firmly held at right angles against the abdominal wall. Because of the bladder's cylindrical rather than spherical shape when distended, an estimate of its size can be obtained by moving a 5.0-MHz linear scanner (field depth of 10 cm) cranially along the ventral midline from the level of the pubic symphysis. The posterior reproductive tract can be imaged by directing the sector transducer toward the tail head from its midline position immediately cranial to the pubic symphysis.

Right Kidney

Examination of the right kidney necessitates shaving the fleece from an area of the right sublumbar fossa immediately caudal to the last rib. The sector transducer head is firmly held against the skin to ensure good visualization of the right kidney juxtaposed the caudal lobe of the liver.

Abomasal Diameter of Neonatal Lambs

The abomasal diameter of neonatal lambs can be measured using a 5- to 6.5-MHz sector scanner applied at right angles to the abdominal wall at the umbilicus. The abomasum can be clearly identified as a hypoechoic area delineated by a hyperechoic wall. The vertical distance is measured between the probe head and the far abomasal wall.

Vaginal Prolapse

The contents of the vaginal prolapse can be readily determined using either linear array or sector scanners.

Scrotum

Sequential examination of the pampiniform plexus, testicle, and tail of the epididymis is undertaken as the linear or sector scanner is moved distally over the lateral aspect of each spermatic cord, testicle, and tail of the epididymis.

Joints

Ultrasonography using a 7.5-MHz linear array scanner with a stand-off can provide some additional useful information regarding the thickness of the joint capsule and extent and nature of any joint effusion. However, such information can more readily be obtained by careful palpation; arthrocentesis often fails because of the presence of a pannus.

ULTRASONOGRAPHIC FINDINGS
Chest

The surface of normal aerated lung (visceral or pulmonary pleura) is characterized by the uppermost white linear echo with equally spaced reverberation artifacts below this line (**Figs. 1** and **2**; Video 1). The chest wall is approximately 1 cm thick in 20- to 40-kg lambs extending up to 3 cm in adult sheep in good body condition with subcutaneous fat and skeletal muscle (80–100 kg; body condition score 3 or greater, scale 1–5). The visceral pleura can be observed moving 2 to 5 mm in a vertical plane during respiration. There is no detectable pleural fluid in normal sheep.

Lung Consolidation

Superficial areas of consolidated lung parenchyma transmit sound waves and appear more hypoechoic than surrounding lung tissue (**Fig. 3**; Video 2). Airways within consolidated lung appear as 3- to 10-mm hyperechoic areas within the hypoechoic lung parenchyma.

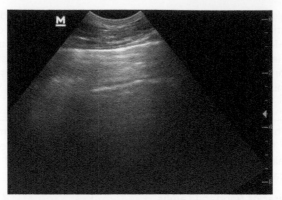

Fig. 1. The surface of normal aerated lung (visceral or pulmonary pleura) is characterized by the uppermost white linear echo with a reverberation artifact below this line. Using a 5-MHz sector scanner, the probe head is at the top of the image, dorsal is to the left, and centimeter markers in the right hand margin.

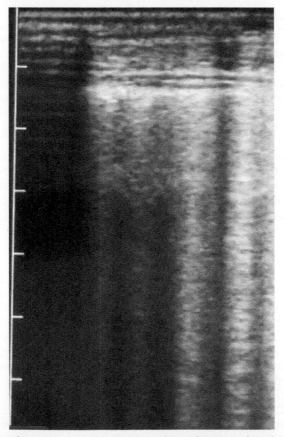

Fig. 2. The surface of normal aerated lung (visceral or pulmonary pleura) is characterized by the uppermost white linear echo. Using a 5-MHz sector scanner, the probe head is at the top of the image, dorsal is to the left, and centimeter markers in the left hand margin.

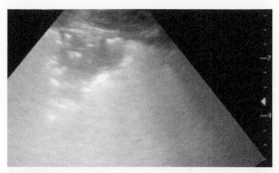

Fig. 3. Using a 5-MHz sector scanner, abrupt loss of the bright linear echo formed by normal aerated lung tissue (visceral or pulmonary pleura) can be seen replaced by a triangular-shaped hypoechoic area representing an OPA lesion.

Pleural Effusion

Pleural effusion transmits sound waves readily and appears as an anechoic area that increases in depth as the probe head travels ventrally down the chest wall, but such pathology is rare in sheep.

Pleural/Lung Abscesses

The white linear echo of the normal visceral pleura is lost with the pleural abscess, appearing as an uniform anechoic area containing many hyperechoic dots caused by gas echoes bordered by a broad hyperechoic line representing the abscess capsule (**Figs. 4** and **5**; Videos 3 and 4). With extensive pleural abscessation/pyo-thorax, where the abscess extends to occupy most of one side of the chest and

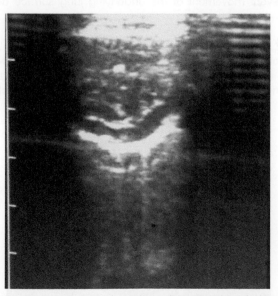

Fig. 4. Using a 5-MHz linear scanner, the 2.5-cm-diameter pleural abscess appears as an anechoic area containing many hyperechoic dots caused by gas echoes bordered by a broad hyperechoic line representing the abscess capsule. Shadowing on either side of the image is caused by the adjacent ribs.

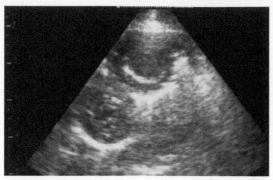

Fig. 5. Using a 5-MHz sector scanner, two pleural/lung abscesses appear as anechoic areas containing many hyperechoic dots caused by gas echoes bordered by broad hyperechoic lines representing the abscess capsule.

contains up to 3 L of pus, auscultation of the lung field may only reveal transmitted gut sounds, particularly rumen contraction sounds when the abscess occupies the left thorax.

Fibrinous Pleurisy

Exudate within the pleural space (**Fig. 6**; Video 5) appears as an anechoic area containing numerous hyperechoic strands (fibrin). There is consolidation of the ventral margin of the lung. In severe cases, unilateral pleurisy may extend for up to 10 cm from the chest wall with a hyperechoic lattice work appearance containing numerous anechoic pockets (**Fig. 7**; Video 6). There is attenuation of lung and heart sounds upon auscultation of the affected side in animals with extensive unilateral lesions. Fibrinous pleurisy may prevent movement of the underlying lung surface during respiratory excursions.

Ovine Pulmonary Adenocarcinoma

The first indication of changes in the superficial lung parenchyma caused by OPA is the abrupt loss of the bright linear echo formed by normal aerated lung tissue (visceral or pulmonary pleura) to be replaced by a large hypoechoic area in the

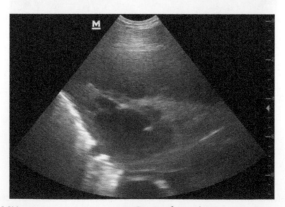

Fig. 6. Using a 5-MHz sector scanner, up to 8 cm of exudate appears as a hypoechoic area between the parietal pleura and bright linear echo, which represents the aerated lung surface (visceral pleura).

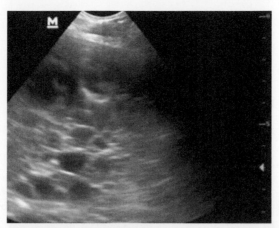

Fig. 7. Using a 5-MHz sector scanner, unilateral pleurisy is seen extending for up to 8 cm from the chest wall with a hyperechoic lattice work appearance containing numerous anechoic pockets.

ventral margins of the lung lobes at the fifth or sixth intercostal spaces (**Figs. 8–10**; Videos 7–9). The hypoechoic areas visualized during ultrasonography, corresponding to lung tissue invaded by tumor cells causing consolidation (**Fig. 11**), allow the extent and distribution of the OPA lesions to be accurately defined during the ultrasonographic examination. Direct comparison of the echogenic appearance of affected right lung with adjacent liver shows the extent of cellular proliferation within the OPA mass (see Video 9). This video is achieved by scanning through affected

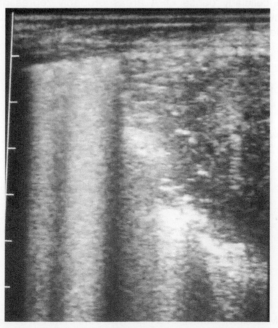

Fig. 8. Using a 5-MHz linear scanner, the sharply demarcated hypoechoic area ventrally corresponds to the distinct OPA tumor.

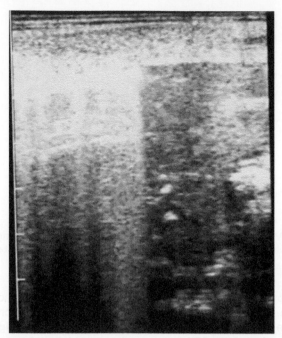

Fig. 9. Using a 5-MHz linear scanner, the large and sharply demarcated (>6 cm deep) hypoechoic area corresponds to consolidated lung tissue invaded by OPA tumor.

lung then diaphragm into the liver. Small focal hyperechoic areas clearly identified within the more cellularly dense OPA areas probably represent large airways. Hyperechoic circular areas measuring 1 to 2 cm in diameter within an OPA mass with distal shadowing probably represent either an abscess or necrotic center (**Figs. 12–14**).

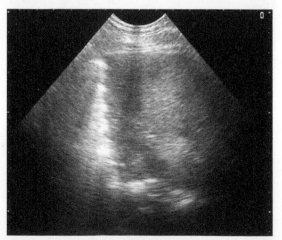

Fig. 10. Using a 5-MHz sector scanner, a vertical hyperechoic line can be seen that represents the distinct separation of the normal hyperechoic visceral pleura dorsally from the hypoechoic mass of the OPA lesion ventrally.

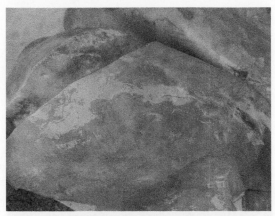

Fig. 11. Necropsy reveals the sharp delineation of normal lung dorsally from the OPA tumour ventrally (see **Figs. 8–10**). Note the sharp demarcation on both the lung surface and on cut section.

Case reports show where the diagnosis of OPA is made using linear and sectors scanners; the sharp demarcation between tumor-affected lung ventrally and normal lung is clearly shown (Videos 10–13).

Fibrinous pleurisy causing adhesions between OPA-affected lung and the pericardial sac is seen ultrasonographically and at necropsy in Video 13; the left lung shows 3 to 4 abscesses measuring 1 to 4 cm in diameter within OPA-affected lung and at necropsy. It proved difficult to separate the pleurae on the left side, and the abscesses are better shown involving the lung once it had been removed from the chest cavity.

HEART
Congenital Cardiac Defects

Congenital cardiac defects[15] and tumors[16] in lambs are rare such that single cases are often reported in the literature.

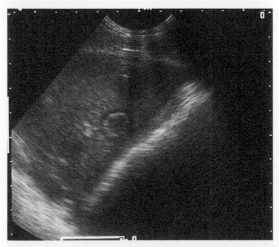

Fig. 12. Using a 5-MHz sector scanner, a 1.5-cm abscess with a distinct capsule within the OPA mass can be seen.

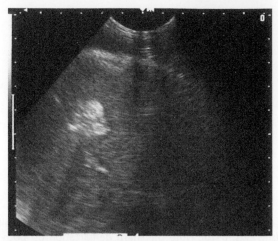

Fig. 13. Using a 5-MHz sector scanner, a 2-cm-diameter hyperechoic lesion with distant shadowing can be seen, which represents a necrotic center within the OPA mass.

Vegetative Endocarditis

Vegetative lesions on the heart valves (vegetative endocarditis) of sheep are generally small and difficult to image, but larger lesions can be imaged with 5- to 6.5-MHz sector scanners (**Figs. 15** and **16**). Color-coded Doppler sonography may be necessary to detect valvular dysfunction caused by smaller heart valve lesions.

Pericarditis

Septic pericarditis is rare in sheep, and diseases causing significant pericardial effusion/exudate generally cause sudden death (such as clostridial diseases) such that ultrasonographic examination of the pericardium is rarely undertaken.

ABDOMEN
Ascites

The scant peritoneal fluid in normal sheep cannot be visualized during ultrasonographic examination. Ascitic fluid appears as an anechoic area with abdominal

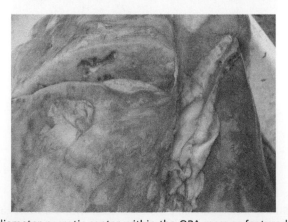

Fig. 14. A 2-cm-diameter necrotic center within the OPA mass as featured in **Fig. 13**.

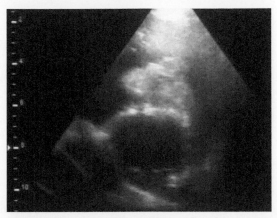

Fig. 15. Using a 5-MHz sector scanner, 2.5-cm-diameter highly irregular hyperechoic mass involving the tricuspid valve is seen. See **Fig. 16**.

viscera displaced dorsally in the standing animal. The intestines are clearly outlined as hyperechoic (bright white) lines/circles containing material of varying echogenicity (**Fig. 17**; Video 14). By maintaining the probe head in the same position for 10 to 20 seconds, digesta can be seen as multiple small dots of varying echogenicity forcibly propelled within the intestines. Accumulation of transudate is seen in sheep with very low serum protein concentrations in diseases such as paratuberculosis but has also been reported in cases of right-sided heart failure caused by bacterial endocarditis. Large amounts of transudate accumulate in sheep with intestinal adenocarcinoma in which transcoelomic spread of the tumor causes impaired lymphatic drainage.

Peritonitis

With the exception of subacute fasciolosis, significant peritoneal exudation is rarely seen in sheep with peritoneal reaction limited by the omentum to focal fibrinous/fibrous adhesions and localized accumulations of peritoneal exudate. Two well-encapsulated

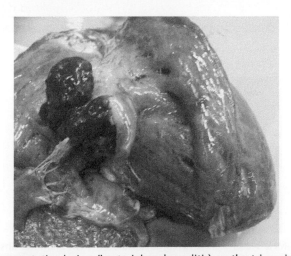

Fig. 16. Irregular vegetative lesion (bacterial endocarditis) on the tricuspid valve.

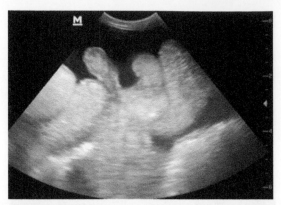

Fig. 17. Using a 5-MHz sector scanner, ascitic fluid can be seen appearing as an anechoic area with intestines displaced dorsally in the standing animal clearly outlined as 1 to 2 diameter hyperechoic circles and longer cylinders containing digesta of varying echogenicity.

abscesses surrounded by omentum are imaged in **Fig. 18** and are shown at necropsy in Video 15; the cause of these abscesses could not be determined.

Small Intestinal Torsion

Torsion of the small intestine around the root of the mesentery is not uncommon. The intestines involved in the torsion are grossly distended with little propulsion of digesta; an increased amount of peritoneal fluid is also seen (Video 16).

Intra-abdominal Hemorrhage

Intra-abdominal hemorrhage most commonly arises either during late pregnancy associated with vaginal prolapse or during unskilled dystocia correction. Hemorrhage results from rupture of blood vessels in the broad ligament and can be imaged with the probe head positioned immediately cranial to the pubis (**Fig. 19**; Video 17).

Liver

The liver is readily identified in the seventh to eleventh intercostal spaces on the right side.

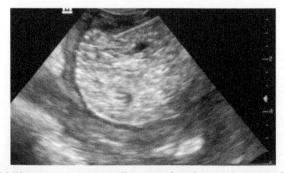

Fig. 18. Using a 5-MHz sector scanner, well-encapsulated 4-cm-diameter abscess can be seen within the abdominal cavity.

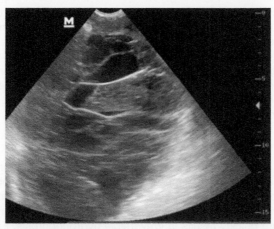

Fig. 19. Intra-abdominal hemorrhage can result from rupture of blood vessels in the broad ligament and is imaged with the probe head positioned immediately cranial to the pubis.

Liver Fluke

The most common liver problem in sheep is liver fluke (predominantly *Fasciola hepatica* infestation). Hepatomegaly and multiple hyperechoic dots within the liver parenchyma (**Fig. 20**; Video 18), representing accumulations of inflammatory cells, are common findings in sheep with subacute fasciolosis.[11] These lesions resolved within 1 month of treatment with triclabendazole.

Loss of normal liver architecture and distension of the gallbladder (Video 19) is commonly seen in chronic liver fluke infestation. Romanski[17] reported gallbladder dimensions measured ultrasonographically in sheep after various intervals during fasting with a doubling of volume after 2 days and suggested that such measurement could provide important clinical information. These data support the necropsy findings of gallbladder distension in cachectic sheep.

Large liver abscesses caused by *Corynebacterium pseudotuberculosis*, the causal agent of caseous lymphadenitis, are not uncommon in many countries including the United States.[18,19] Where infection does cause large liver abscesses, these lesions should be readily identified during ultrasonographic examination.

Ultrasonographic examination of the liver has confirmed the presence of ovine hydatid cysts and the potential use of ultrasonography as a mass screening approach

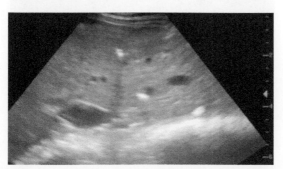

Fig. 20. Using a 5-MHz sector scanner, multiple hyperechoic dots can be seen throughout the liver parenchyma with shadowing that represents accumulations of inflammatory cells in a sheep with subacute fasciolosis.

for cystic echinococcosis.[20,21] Cysts of *Echinococcus granulosus* in the liver of sheep were located by ultrasonography and injected with dipeptide methyl ester and the treatment response monitored ultrasonographically.[22]

Although hepatocellular tumors are not uncommon in old sheep, such lesions are usually only recognized at the slaughter plant in ewes culled for poor condition; however, it was reported that liver tissue obtained via ultrasound-guided percutaneous liver biopsy suggested n diagnosis of adenocarcinoma of the liver, which was later confirmed at necropsy.[23]

URINARY TRACT

Ultrasonographic examination of the bladder and caudal abdomen provides useful information in male sheep with suspected partial or complete urethral obstruction (Video 20), which is a common condition of intensively reared rams.[24] Early recognition of clinical signs by the owner and prompt veterinary treatment are essential because urinary back pressure quickly results in irreversible hydronephrosis. Early diagnosis of urolithiasis allows prompt surgical correction of breeding rams by tube cystotomy[25] (**Fig. 21**; Video 21) and rapid implementation of control measures to prevent further cases.

Examination using a 5.0-MHz linear array scanner readily identifies distended bladder and uroperitoneum if present, but the true size of the bladder may not be measured because it may extend to 20 cm in diameter, thereby exceeding the 10-cm field of many linear array scanners. The distended bladder extends 6 to 8 cm in diameter cranial to the pelvic brim in 20- to 40-kg growing lambs and 12 to 16 cm diameter in mature rams (**Figs. 22** and **23**). The bladder wall appears as a hyperechoic circle; edema of the wall results in widening of this white line. In those rams with uroperitoneum, fibrin tags can sometimes be seen as fine hyperechoic filaments with the anechoic fluid.

Urinary tract infections leading to pyelonephritis are rare in sheep with the exception of those males that have undergone subischial urethrostomy surgery to bypass the site of obstructive urolithiasis. In cases of cystitis, the bladder wall appears much thicker than normal with fibrin tags on the mucosal surface that appear as hyperechoic strands. Large fibrin clots, typically represented by irregularly shaped hypoechoic circles containing hyperechoic dots, are often present within the distended bladder.

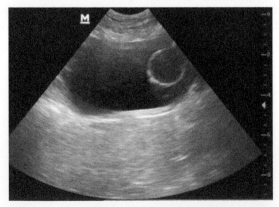

Fig. 21. Tube cystotomy surgery used for the treatment of obstructive urolithiasis in a ram. The inflated cuff of the Foley catheter is visible as a 2-cm-diameter hyperechoic circle within the bladder, which measures approximately 4 cm. A 5-MHz sector scanner was used.

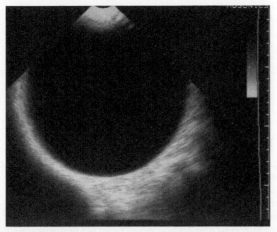

Fig. 22. The distended urinary bladder extends to greater than 12 cm diameter (see **Fig. 23**).

Kidney

Examination of the right kidney is undertaken using a 5.0-MHz sector transducer; the concave nature of the right sublumbar fossae prevents good contact and use of a linear transducer. The right kidney is juxtaposed to the caudal pole of the liver underlying the dorsal aspect of the right sublumbar fossa (**Fig. 24**). Advanced hydronephrosis can be identified by the grossly increased renal pelvis, which is represented by the anechoic (fluid-filled) center of the kidney (**Figs. 25** and **26**; Video 22). It is not always possible to scan the left kidney in sheep via the flank, but such examination is not necessary because the urinary tract obstruction is distal to the ureters; therefore, the condition affects both kidneys equally.

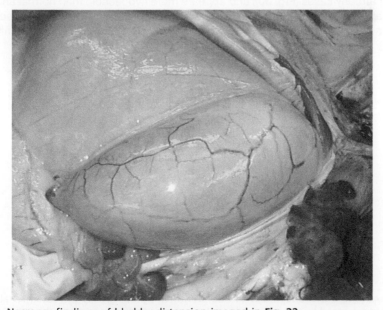

Fig. 23. Necropsy findings of bladder distension imaged in **Fig. 22**.

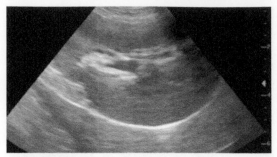

Fig. 24. Ultrasonographic appearance of a normal right kidney. The renal capsule appears as the convex hyperechoic line.

Biricik and colleagues[26] concluded from their studies on young lambs with obstructive urolithiaisis that B-mode and color-coded Doppler sonography might provide useful information for detection of changes in kidneys, like hydronephrosis, renal swelling, and elevated resistance in the renal interlobar artery. A large, greater-than-10-cm diameter renal carcinoma is shown in Video 23 and **Figs. 27** and **28**.

SCROTUM

The normal testicle appears as a uniform hypoechoic area with the hyperechoic mediastinum often visible. The tail of the epididymis is distinct from the testicle and considerably smaller in diameter (2–3 cm compared with >7 cm) with a distinct capsule.

Testicular Atrophy

The testicle(s) is much reduced in size (normal, >7 cm in diameter (**Fig. 29**), frequently 5 cm for atrophy cases (**Fig. 30**)) and appears more hypoechoic than normal and contains many hyperechoic dots. These hyperechoic dots are thought to represent the fibrous supporting architecture now more obvious after atrophy of the seminiferous

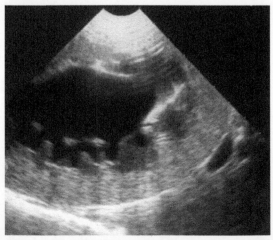

Fig. 25. Advanced hydronephrosis can be identified by the grossly increased renal pelvis which is represented by the enlarged anechoic center of the kidney (see **Fig. 26**).

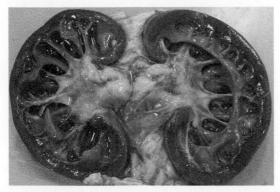

Fig. 26. Necropsy findings of the hydronephrotic kidney featured in **Fig. 25**.

tubules. Ultrasonography was reported to be useful for the diagnosis of intrascrotal abnormalities after experimental inoculation with *Trueperella pyogenes* into the testicle, especially during investigation of chronic disease after clinical findings had subsided.[27]

Epididymitis

Epididymitis caused by *Brucella ovis* and *Actinobacillus seminis/Histophilus ovis* is a major cause of ram infertility in many countries. Ultrasonographic examination in rams with epididymitis finds a normal pampiniform plexus. Typically, the swollen scrotal contents frequently appear as multiple 1- to 5-cm diameter anechoic areas containing many bright spots surrounded by broad hyperechoic lines (fibrous capsule) extending up to 1 cm in thickness typical of chronic abscesses. The abscesses generally involve the tail of the epididymis but may extend to involve the body and head. The testicle is embedded within fibrous tissue reaction and is much reduced in size. The testicle appears more hypoechoic than normal and contains many hyperechoic spots consistent with testicular atrophy.[28] In unilateral epididymitis cases, the contralateral testicle is much smaller than normal and appears more hypoechoic.

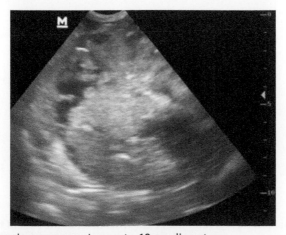

Fig. 27. A renal carcinoma measuring up to 10 cm diameter.

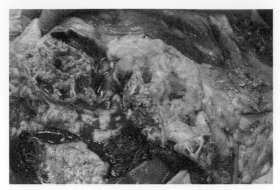

Fig. 28. A renal carcinoma measuring up to 10 cm diameter at necropsy.

PREGNANCY

Real time transrectal ultrasonographic scanning of sheep between days 24 and 34 of gestation offers a safe, accurate, and practical means for diagnosing pregnancy.[29] Accuracies of diagnosis of pregnancy of more than 99%; of differentiation of barren, single-, and multiple-bearing ewes of 98%; and of determination of actual fetal numbers of 97% can be achieved in practice at scanning rates of at least 1 ewe per minute.[4]

Obstetric Problems

Ultrasonographic examination is of particular value where transabdominal ballotment suggests the presence of a fetus in utero after delivery of lamb(s) some 12 to 48 hours previously, but contraction of the cervix prevents further manual examination of the uterus. It can prove difficult to differentiate the contracted uterus from a uterine horn containing a single lamb by transabdominal ballotment alone, but this problem can be easily resolved by ultrasonographic examination of the caudal abdomen (Video 24).

Ultrasonography has been used to monitor uterine involution postpartum, which was delayed in ewes after manual correction of dystocia and cesarean section.[30]

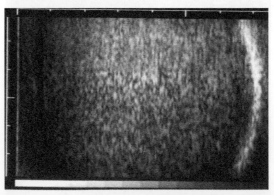

Fig. 29. The normal testicle is greater than 7 cm in diameter at the start of the breeding season in mature rams.

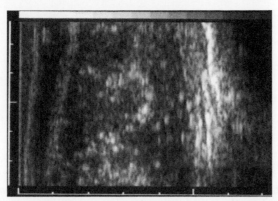

Fig. 30. With atrophy the testicle is often less than 5 cm in diameter and appears more hypoechoic than normal and may contain many hyperechoic dots (see **Fig. 29**).

Uterine Torsion

Uterine torsion is a problematic diagnosis in sheep because vaginal examination is restricted by the narrow diameter of the reproductive tract and will not identify a torsion involving the body of the uterus cranial to the cervix. A recent article described the application of transabdominal ultrasound examination of the uterine wall as close to the cervix as possible (ventral midline immediately cranial to the pelvic brim with the probe head directed vertically) as a noninvasive means of detecting uterine torsion in sheep.[31] Edema of the uterine wall after torsion resulted in a doubling of the thickness from 5 mm to more than 10 mm. Although a 7.5-MHz scanner was used in this investigation, a 5-MHz linear scanner should provide diagnostic quality sonograms. In the case of uterine torsion seen by this author, the lamb was 1 month overdue based on the single artificial insemination date; the cotyledons were poorly defined and the fetal fluids were not anechoic (**Fig. 31**). This image looks to be of poor quality but this is because of autolysis (**Fig. 32**).

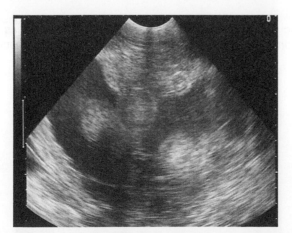

Fig. 31. In this case of a 720° uterine torsion, the cotyledons are very poorly defined, and the fetal fluids are not distinctly anechoic. The quality of this sonogram should be judged alongside the necropsy findings (see **Fig. 32**) where the uterine wall, placenta, and single lamb are autolytic; the uterine wall is green with widespread fibrin on the serosal surface.

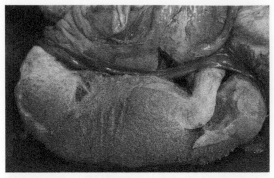

Fig. 32. Necropsy findings of the uterus imaged in **Fig. 31**; the uterine wall, placenta, and single lamb are autolytic; there is widespread and organized fibrin on the serosal surface of the uterus.

Pyometra is uncommon in sheep but can be identified ultrasonographically with the uterine horns distended 6 to 8 cm with pus (**Fig. 33**). Uterine tumors are rare in sheep, but cases of leiomyomas have been identified in sheep presenting in poor body condition (**Figs. 34** and **35**).

VAGINAL PROLAPSE

Vaginal prolapse may comprise dorsal vaginal wall, urinary bladder, uterine horn(s), or both urinary bladder and uterine horn(s). Urinary bladder is readily identified as an anechoic (black) area on the sonogram usually greater than 8 cm in diameter and compressed dorsoventrally (**Fig. 36**). A fold in the bladder wall, which presents as a hyperechoic (white) line, can often be visualized in the ventral one-third of the anechoic area. Sections through the tips of uterine horn(s) appear as anechoic circles measuring 3 to 5 cm in diameter bordered by the hyperechoic uterine wall; caruncles are not usually observed.

UDDER

Ultrasonographic examination of an udder with palpable abscesses (Video 25) has limited application in clinical practice. Ultrasonographic measurements of the length

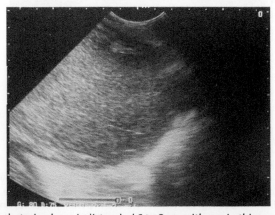

Fig. 33. The imaged uterine horn is distended 6 to 8 cm with pus in this example of pyometra.

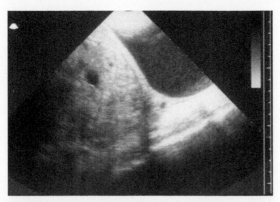

Fig. 34. Leiomyoma measuring up to 16 cm positioned dorsal to the 7 cm diameter urinary bladder (see **Fig. 35**).

and width of the teat canal in lactating ewes seemed to be positively correlated to the California mastitis test results leading the authors to conclude that ultrasonography holds promise for the future in evaluating the health of the udder of small ruminants.[32,33]

JOINTS

Arthrosonography of sheep with chronic arthritis/synovitis found gross thickening of the joint capsule visible ultrasonographically as a hyperechoic band up to 20 mm thick,[8] but such a condition can readily be determined by careful palpation.

MUSCLE

Ultrasonography could not be used for quantitative assessment of post-injection muscle damage where creatine kinase assay provided a more accurate evaluation of macroscopic muscle damage.[34]

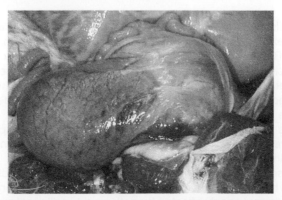

Fig. 35. Necropsy findings of the sonogram featured in **Fig. 34**. The cadaver is positioned in dorsal recumbency with a ventral midline approach at necropsy; the leiomyoma is dorsal to the urinary bladder.

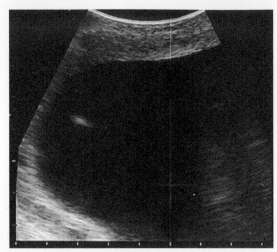

Fig. 36. Urinary bladder in the vaginal prolapse is readily identified as an anechoic (*black*) area usually greater than 8 cm in diameter and compressed dorsoventrally.

ABOMASUM IN NEONATES

Perinatal lamb mortality, defined as losses within the first 3 days of life, is the major cause of lamb deaths with estimates ranging from 10 to 25%.[35–37] Ultrasonographic examination of the abomasum of neonatal lambs provides an immediate indication to the veterinary investigator whether lambs have sucked. The difference in lamb abomasal diameter before and after sucking is so large, 3 cm versus 8 to 10 cm, that minor errors in individual lamb recordings should not affect the collection of meaningful data from 20 or more lambs and their interpretation.

BRAIN

Ultrasound scan has been used as an aid to *Coenurus cerebralis* cyst localization in a lamb.[38]

DISCUSSION

In addition to assisting the veterinarian establish a specific diagnosis at the time of the first ultrasound examination, repeated examinations allow the lesion(s) to be monitored over time. Recording ultrasound findings either as still images or videos also allows full review should treatment prove unsuccessful when it is essential to critically evaluate interpretations of the ultrasound recordings when the pathologic condition is revealed at necropsy. This practice has been adopted in the video recordings in this article where possible.

In the author's experience of farm animal practice, ultrasonography is especially useful in the investigation of respiratory diseases in both cattle and sheep and in obstructive urolithiasis in male sheep.

Respiratory disease is common in sheep, but it proves difficult to diagnose specific diseases/lesions by clinical examination alone because the respiratory rate and intensity of lung sounds are variably affected by gathering, handling stresses, body condition score, and painful lesions. It may prove difficult to distinguish wheezes and crackles, and not all experts agree on what they hear and what pathologic changes those sounds represent.[2] Indeed, in many respiratory diseases, breath sounds are markedly attenuated or absent. Ultrasonographic examination of the chest allows critical evaluation of the pleurae and establishment of a definitive diagnosis in most cases. The increasing availability of sector scanners in sheep practice offers exciting diagnostic opportunities. Indeed, the clinical application of ultrasound examination of the equine chest was reported almost 25 years ago.[39]

The role of ultrasonography in the logical approach to a novel situation is illustrated in the diagnosis of pelvic nerve paralysis in 2 rams.[40] Marked urinary bladder distension, hydroureters, severe bilateral hydronephrosis, and perirenal fluid accumulation were identified ultrasonographically. Both rams were observed to pass a free flow of urine, but the flow rate was less than normal, and the duration was reduced to around 5 to 10 seconds when around 20 to 30 seconds is considered normal. There was normal tail and rectal muscle tone and normal perineal and pelvic limb reflexes. Detailed dissection at necropsy found no evidence of urethral obstruction. These cases warranted more detailed investigation because the rams passed a free flow of urine and not just occasional drops of urine, which is the classical presentation of urethral obstruction. Without the ultrasound findings at the time of clinical examination, the diagnosis of pelvic nerve paralysis may have been overlooked.

SUPPLEMENTARY DATA

Supplementary data related to this article can be found online at http://dx.doi.org/10.1016/j.cvfa.2015.09.008.

REFERENCES

1. Cousens C, Graham M, Sales J, et al. Evaluation of the efficacy of clinical diagnosis of ovine pulmonary adenocarcinoma. Vet Rec 2008;162:88–90.
2. Scott PR, Collie DDS, McGorum B, et al. Relationship between thoracic auscultation and lung pathology detected by ultrasonography in sheep. Vet J 2010;186: 53–7.
3. Fowler DG, Wilkins JF. Diagnosis of pregnancy and number of foetuses in sheep by real time ultrasound imaging. 1: effect of number of foetuses, stage of gestation, operator, and breed of ewe on accuracy of diagnosis. Livest Prod Sci 1984; 11:437–40.
4. White R, Russel IR, Fowler DG. Real-time ultrasonic scanning in the diagnosis of pregnancy and the determination of fetal numbers in sheep. Vet Rec 1984;115: 140–3.
5. Russel A. Nutrition of the pregnant ewe. In Pract 1985;7:23–9.
6. Scott PR, Gessert ME, Marsh D. Ultrasonographic measurement of the abomasum of neonatal lambs. Vet Rec 1997;141:524–5.
7. Scott PR, Gessert ME. Ultrasonographic examination of the ovine thorax. Vet J 1998;155:305–10.
8. Macrae A, Scott PR. The normal ultrasonographic appearance of ovine joints and the uses of arthrosonography in the evaluation of chronic ovine joint disease. Vet J 1999;158:135–43.
9. Scott PR. Ultrasonographic examination of the urinary tract of sheep. In Pract 2000;22:329–34.
10. Scott PR, Gessert ME. Application of ultrasonographic examination of the ovine foetus in normal sheep and those presenting with obstetrical problems. Vet J 2000;159:291–2.

11. Scott PR, Sargison ND, Macrae AI, et al. An outbreak of subacute fasciolosis in soay sheep: biochemical, histological and ultrasonographic studies. Vet J 2005; 170:325–31.
12. Scott PR, Gessert ME. Ultrasonographic examination of 12 ovine vaginal prolapses. Vet J 1998;155:323–4.
13. Braun U, Schefer U, Fohn J. Urinary tract ultrasonography in normal rams and in rams with obstructive urolithiasis. Can Vet J 1992;33:654–9.
14. Braun U, Schefer U, Gerber D. Ultrasonography of the urinary tract of female sheep. Am J Vet Res 1992;53:1734–9.
15. Sameluk N, Reif S, Skrodzki M, et al. Persistent ductus arteriosus (PDA) and atrial septum defect (ASD) in a lamb. A case report. Tierarztl Prax 2003;31:204–20.
16. Braun U, Hagen A, Pusterla N, et al. Echocardiographic diagnosis of a cardiac fibrosarcoma in the right atrium of a sheep. Schweiz Arch Tierheilkd 1995;137: 187–92.
17. Romanski KW. Ultrasonographic monitoring of gallbladder dynamics during fasting and feeding conditions in sheep. Acta Vet 2004;73:29–35.
18. Stoops SG, Renshaw HW, Thilstead JP. Ovine caseous lymphadenitis: disease prevalence, lesion distribution, and thoracic manifestation in a population of mature cull sheep from western United States. Am J Vet Res 1984;40:1110–4.
19. Gnad DP, Van Metre DC, Angelos SM, et al. Diagnosing weight loss in sheep: a practical approach. Compend Contin Educ Vet 2000;22:S16–23.
20. Guarnera EA, Zanzottera EM, Pereya H, et al. Ultrasonographic diagnosis of ovine cystic echinococcosis. Vet Radiol Ultrasound 2001;42:352–4.
21. Lahmara S, Ben Chéhidab F, Pétavyc AF, et al. Ultrasonographic screening for cystic echinococcosis in sheep in Tunisia. Vet Parasitol 2007;143:42–9.
22. Lahmara S, Sarciron ME, Chehida FB. Cystic hydatic disease in sheep: treatment with percutaneous aspiration and injection with dipeptide methyl ester. Vet Res Commun 2006;30:379–91.
23. Lofstedt J, Schelling S, Stowater J, et al. Antemortem diagnosis of hepatic adenocarcinoma in a ewe. J Am Vet Med Assoc 1988;193:1537–8.
24. Angus KW. Diseases of the urinary tract. In: Martin WB, Aitken ID, editors. Diseases of sheep. Oxford (United Kingdom): Blackwell Science; 2000. p. 344–51.
25. Cockcroft PD. Dissolution of obstructive urethral urolithiasis in a ram. Vet Rec 1993;132:486–7.
26. Biricik HS, Cimtay I, Ozuturk A, et al. B-Mode and colour coded doppler sonography of kidneys in lambs with urolithiasis and in healthy lambs. Dtsch Tierarztl Wochenschr 2003;110:502–5.
27. Gouletsou PG, Fthenakis GC, Cripps PJ. Experimentally induced orchitis associated with Arcanobacterium pyogenes: clinical, ultrasonographic, seminological and pathological features. Theriogenology 2004;62:1307–18.
28. Karaca F, Aksoy M, Kaya A, et al. Spermatic granuloma in the ram: diagnosis by ultrasonography and semen characteristics. Vet Radiol Ultrasound 1999;40: 402–6.
29. Garcia A, Neary MK, Kelly GR, et al. Accuracy of ultrasonography in early pregnancy diagnosis in the ewe. Theriogenology 1993;39:847–61.
30. Hauser B, Bostedt H. Ultrasonographic observations of the uterine regression in the ewe under different obstetrical conditions. J Vet Med A Physiol Pathol Clin Med 2002;49:511–6.
31. Wehrend A, Bostedt H, Burkhardt E. The use of trans-abdominal B mode ultrasonography to diagnose intra-partum uterine torsion in the ewe. Vet J 2002;176: 69–70.

32. Franz S, Hofmann-Parisot M, Baumgartner W, et al. Ultrasonography of the teat canal in cows and sheep. Vet Rec 2001;149:109–12.
33. Franz S, Hoffman-Parisot M, Gutler S. Clinical and ultrasonographic findings in the mammary gland of sheep. N Z Vet J 2003;51:238–43.
34. Ferre PJ, Concordet D, Laroute V, et al. Comparison of ultrasonography and pharmacokinetic analysis of creatine kinase release for quantitative assessment of postinjection muscle damage. Am J Vet Res 2001;62:1698–705.
35. Eales FA, Gilmour JS, Barlow RM, et al. Causes of hypothermia in 89 lambs. Vet Rec 1982;110:118–20.
36. Barlow RM, Gardiner AC, Angus KW, et al. Clinical, biochemical and pathological study of perinatal lambs in a commercial flock. Vet Rec 1987;120:357–63.
37. Hindson JC, Winter AC. Outline of clinical diagnosis in sheep. Sevenoaks (United Kingdom): Wiley Blackwell; 1990. p. 62.
38. Doherty ML, McAllister H, Healy A. Ultrasound as an aid to coenurus cerebralis cyst localisation in a lamb. Vet Rec 1989;124:591–2.
39. Reef VB, Boy MG, Reid CF, et al. Comparison between diagnostic ultrasonography and radiography in the evaluation of horses and cattle with thoracic disease: 56 cases (1984-1985). J Am Vet Med Assoc 1991;198:2112–8.
40. Scott PR. Clinical, ultrasonographic and pathological description of bladder distension with consequent hydroureters, severe hydronephrosis and perirenal fluid accumulation in two rams putatively ascribed to pelvic nerve dysfunction. Small Ruminant Research 2012;107:45–8.

Ultrasound Use for Body Composition and Carcass Quality Assessment in Cattle and Lambs

Richard Gregory Tait Jr, MS, PhD, PAS (Professional Animal Scientist)

KEYWORDS

- Beef quality • Body composition • Genetic improvement • Lamb quality
- Longissimus • Marbling • Ultrasound

KEY POINTS

- Ultrasound-measured body composition traits in seed stock have high genetic correlations (≥ 0.5) with carcass traits in harvested animals.
- Beef seed stock producers have demonstrated tremendous adoption of ultrasound technology to evaluate seed stock animals for body composition traits.
- The Ultrasound Guidelines Council certifications provide confidence to beef producers that technicians collecting and processing their ultrasound images are well qualified.
- Ultrasound body composition evaluation in beef and lambs for genetic improvement is a coordinated effort between the producer and the ultrasound technician.

INTRODUCTION

Carcass traits in harvested beef animals are economically relevant traits[1] (ERTs) because they are used to quantify the economic value of an animal to processors and subsequently to consumers. Carcass traits such as hot carcass weight, 12th rib subcutaneous fat thickness, 12th rib longissimus area, and 12th rib marbling are all important attributes to red meat yield and anticipated consumer acceptability of the product.[2] Up until the mid 1990s, the characterization of a seed stock animal for their carcass traits was limited to a pedigree estimate of an animal's expected progeny differences (EPDs). The pedigree estimated EPDs were based on structured sire evaluations designed and managed by breed associations to collect steer progeny

Disclosure statement: Dr R.G. Tait is a member of the board of directors for the Ultrasound Guidelines Council, a nonprofit subcommittee of the US Beef Breeds Council.
Genetics, Breeding, and Animal Health Research Unit, USDA, ARS, US Meat Animal Research Center, PO Box 166, 844 Rd 313, Clay Center, NE 68933, USA
E-mail address: jr.tait@ars.usda.gov

carcass data for evaluation. Often sires were old (>5 years) by the time these evaluations provided information that influenced carcass trait EPDs on the sire and his relatives.

Stouffer and colleagues[3] performed early investigations into the capacity of ultrasound as a tool to measure carcass traits in cattle. The general conclusion was that the development and refinement of the techniques was warranted.[3] Important refinements for the application of ultrasound in beef cattle carcass trait evaluation have occurred in the past 30 years. Those include the availability of (1) brightness mode ultrasound machines[4] and (2) 17.2-cm and larger linear array transducers to measure the cross-sectional longissimus area.[5] Furthermore, research performed in the 1990s demonstrated the utility of ultrasound-measured body composition traits for predicting retail product yield.[6–8]

Utilization of ultrasound for body composition evaluation in seed stock beef cattle increased dramatically after a research project demonstrating the concept of centralized ultrasound processing.[9] In that project, ultrasound images were collected by qualified ultrasound technicians; the images were submitted to a centralized ultrasound processing laboratory; laboratory technicians evaluated the image quality and interpreted the images from acceptable images; data were submitted to beef breed associations; breed associations adjusted the data; breed associations provided raw measures, adjusted measures, and within-contemporary-group ratios back to the producers. Through this research project, it was demonstrated that ultrasound measures of body composition traits (12th rib subcutaneous fat thickness, 12th rib longissimus area, and 12th rib intramuscular fat) in seed stock bulls measured at yearling time had high genetic correlations ($r_g \geq 0.71$) with the analogous carcass traits (12th rib subcutaneous fat, 12th rib longissimus area, and 12th rib marbling) measured in harvested steers.[9] Development of a centralized interpretation laboratory was a huge transition from the previous approach whereby an ultrasound technician interpreted their own images and reported the data back to the breeder and then the breeder chose whether to submit the data to the breed association or not.

At one point beef breeders had ultrasound body composition trait EPDs and carcass trait EPDs available for selection. However, to limit confusion and report on the ERT basis, most breed associations now report carcass EPDs and include the ultrasound body composition traits as indicator traits with high genetic correlations in the carcass trait EPD calculation. More recent evaluations use genetic correlations ($0.52 < r_g < 0.90$) of sex-specific ultrasound body composition traits to steer carcass traits.[10] **Table 1** highlights the differences between carcass traits measured in harvested progeny and ultrasound-measured body composition traits measured in seed stock for carcass trait EPD calculation.

INDICATIONS/CONTRAINDICATIONS

Most beef breed associations in North America have policies limiting ultrasound body composition data for carcass trait EPD calculation to only ultrasound data collected and processed by technicians who are certified by the Ultrasound Guidelines Council (UGC). The UGC Web site (www.ultrasoundbeef.com) maintains lists of (1) accredited laboratories for processing of ultrasound images, (2) certified field technicians who collect the ultrasound images, and (3) ultrasound technologies approved for collection of ultrasound-measured body composition traits. Beyond the publicly displayed lists of field technicians and approved ultrasound technologies, the UGC also conducts the laboratory technician certifications and identifies

Table 1
Comparison of traditional (before ~2000) carcass-measured traits and ultrasound-measured traits of body composition to support seed stock evaluation and selection for improved carcass quality in beef cattle

Attribute	Carcass-Measured Traits	Ultrasound-Measured Traits
Source of data	Structured sire evaluation progeny, usually steers	Self; bull, heifer, or steer acceptable
EPD calculation model	Sire model, ignored dam genetic contributions	Animal model, uses full genetic relationships; included as a correlated trait for carcass trait EPDs
Management considerations	Coordination from breeding commercial cows, through calving cows, feeding progeny, and collection of carcass data at harvest	Animals already being managed in contemporary groups for yearling performance evaluation
Age when own data influences EPD estimate	Minimum 3.5 y, usually 5–6 y	10–15 mo
Rate of adoption[11]	Mid 1970s to 2000 (~25 y) 60,000 records	1998–2000 (3 y) 86,000 records
Current records inventory[12]	104,000	1,578,000
Trait relationships to ERT	The ERT	High genetic correlations (≥ 0.7)[9] to the ERT

proficient laboratory technicians who assess image quality and perform interpretations within the laboratories.

Certification Requirements (Equipment and Technician)

Because ultrasound evaluation of beef seed stock animals for body composition traits is performed at 10 to 15 months of age, but assessment of the accuracy of those measurements and the selections made may not be available until years later, ultrasound technologies contributing data to beef breed associations have been through rigorous system evaluations by the UGC. Any introduction of new ultrasound systems, image capturing systems, or interpretation software and/or gain settings adjustments are all subjected to a system evaluation and approval by the UGC before they are used in beef breed association carcass trait EPD calculations.

Beef seed stock evaluation of body composition traits use UGC-certified field technicians to collect ultrasound images with UGC-approved ultrasound systems and image-capturing software. The images are submitted to UGC-accredited laboratories where UGC-certified laboratory technicians evaluate image quality and provide image interpretations and measures of ultrasound-measured beef carcass traits. An additional process has been developed whereby some UGC field technicians have went through UGC laboratory certification and can use specific software to perform interpretations on site and have the data eligible to be submitted to breed associations.

UGC field technician certification is typically valid for 2 years at a time. There is an absentia field technician certification process developed by the UGC whereby a field technician does not have to participate in the field certification if they meet several criteria:

- Successfully passed multiple field certification evaluations
- Scan a defined number of animals each year they have been certified
- Achieve a defined image quality standard on all of the cattle they have scanned during the previous certification period

Expectations of Producer/Prescanning Management of the Animal

Animals to be evaluated for body composition traits with ultrasound need to be previously identified at the breed association. (This identification usually includes the birth date, parentage, preweaning management group, and preweaning performance information.) Lists of animals with owner and animal identification information are available to the producer from the breed association to ensure correct identification of the animal at the time of scanning. This practice enables merging of the ultrasound body composition trait data to all other performance data on the animal for genetic evaluation purposes. Producers need to ensure all (or as many as possible) animals are within the breed association's acceptable age window for ultrasound evaluation on the day ultrasound scanning takes place. Also, the producer needs to know the postweaning management contemporary group for each animal at time of ultrasound scanning so comparisons are representative of the management applied to the animals.

Application of Ultrasound for Carcass Traits in Beef Feedlot Settings

Ultrasound evaluation of body composition has also been implemented in beef feedlot settings.[13,14] Technician certification is not required for feedlot applications of ultrasound evaluation of body composition. Applications of ultrasound for body composition evaluation in feedlots include (1) sorting animals near marketing to identify animals that have achieved specific fat thickness or marbling targets and (2) sorting animals near feedlot entry or at reimplant time into specified outcome groups or management schemes, whereby the goal would be to not sort animals later as they are ready to be marketed. This application of ultrasound to evaluate body composition in the feedlot is best implemented with a chute-side animal assessment and immediate sorting strategy. Both studies[13,14] documented increased accuracy of ultrasound measures compared with carcass data of harvested animals as the ultrasound measures were collected closer to the harvest date versus predictions made 100 days or more before harvest. Additionally, both studies[13,14] reported that logarithmic subcutaneous fat deposition was a better predictor than linear subcutaneous fat deposition predictions, with groups of animals averaging greater than 0.3 cm of subcutaneous fat at prediction time[13] also having an advantage over leaner groups of animals in prediction accuracy of fat deposition. Therefore, application of ultrasound for body composition evaluation in the feedlot needs to occur after the animals have been on feed long enough to express differences for subcutaneous fat deposition to be able to predict outcome groups or subcutaneous-fat-thickness–based optimum harvest dates. The feedlot operator will have an assessment of whether the ultrasound and sorting activity increased returns within a few months. The feedlot operator's assessment will be within a dynamic system based on whether (1) the fed cattle market is increasing or decreasing, (2) the value of more marbling (choice-select spread) is increasing or decreasing, (3) efficiency of gain is improved after ultrasound sorting of animals, and (4) penalties received for marketing overfinished animals were reduced.

Lamb Industry to Beef Industry Comparison on the Use of Ultrasound for Body Composition Traits

Overall, evaluation of lamb body composition with ultrasound is based on similar concepts to the beef industry approach. Evaluation of seed stock animals with ultrasound allows for reduced generation interval and more direct sources of information than sire progeny tests of harvest animals. Like the beef industry, lamb evaluation is based on ultrasound capacity to give accurate measures of subcutaneous fat thickness and longissimus muscle between the 12th and 13th thoracic vertebrae.[15] As shown in **Table 2**, there are differences in these specific measures: (1) fat thickness is measured in a different location, (2) longissimus depth is used to represent lean muscle mass rather than longissimus area, and (3) body composition trait EPDs for seed stock animals are reported in lambs rather than the harvested progeny carcass trait basis.[16] Similar to cattle, acquiring the cross-sectional ultrasound image between the 12th and 13th thoracic vertebrae is a challenge, especially with the vertebrae closer to each other in lambs at typical ultrasound evaluation weights and ages.

TECHNIQUE/PROCEDURE
Patient Positioning and Preparation

The animal should be restrained in a working chute. It is very desirable to have a squeeze chute whereby the sides of the chute can restrain and control the animal and prevent the animal from dropping to its knees where it could choke. Preparation of the scanning sites (**Fig. 1**) is very important for good acoustical contact and consistent comparisons among animals within the contemporary group. To ensure consistency, the hair is to be clipped to less than 1.27 cm in the area of scanning. Then the area should be combed and/or have any dirt and debris blown from the scanning location with air. After cleaning, apply vegetable or canola oil as an acoustical couplant. In cases whereby the ambient temperature is less than 7°C while scanning, supplemental heat should be applied to the acoustical couplant oil and

Table 2
Comparison of beef cattle ultrasound evaluation of body composition traits and lamb ultrasound evaluation of body composition traits

Attribute	Beef Cattle Evaluation	Lamb Evaluation[16]
12th Rib fat thickness measure	Three-fourths lateral distance of longissimus from spine	One-half lateral distance of longissimus from spine
12th Rib muscling measure	Longissimus cross-sectional area	Longissimus depth at deepest point
Additional indicators of fatness	Rump fat thickness	None
Quality assessment	Intramuscular fat percentage	None
Adjustment basis	Age	Weight
Reporting basis of genetic predictions	Steer progeny carcass trait basis	Seed stock ultrasound body composition trait basis

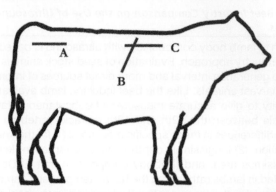

Fig. 1. Approximate locations for ultrasound scanning beef cattle carcass traits. (A) Rump image position: approximately parallel with the spine, in line from the hooks to the pins; rump fat depth is measured from this image. (B) The 12th to 13th rib cross-sectional image of longissimus muscle: parallel between the 12th and 13th thoracic vertebrae; 12th rib subcutaneous fat thickness and 12th rib longissimus area are measured from this image. (C) Intramuscular fat image: longitudinal transducer position nearly parallel with the spine with image showing the longissimus over the 13th thoracic vertebrae, 12th thoracic vertebrae, and usually the 11th thoracic vertebrae. (*From* Wilson DE, Rouse GH. Beef cattle real-time ultrasound scanning guide. Iowa State University Department of Animal Science; 2002; with permission.)

ultrasound equipment. Individual animal weights need to be collected within 7 days of the ultrasound scanning for reporting to the breed association with the ultrasound data.

Initial setup of ultrasound equipment, verification of gain settings, and confirmation of ultrasound images being saved to the image capturing system are critical steps to ensuring a successful scanning session. Furthermore, frequent checks on the ultrasound equipment settings throughout the scan session are also warranted, because incorrect gain settings are cause to reject intramuscular fat images.

Approach

The approach is to approximate the carcass measures collected in harvest facilities (ie, 12th rib subcutaneous fat thickness, 12th rib longissimus area, and 12th rib marbling) or acquire informative, highly repeatable measures for retail product prediction (ie, rump fat thickness).

Specific Technique/Procedure

Consistency in the image collection process is advantageous to establish habits whereby all images are routinely collected and the animal-to-animal comparisons are as consistent as possible for the assessment of body composition traits.

1. Rump fat image is typically the easiest image to collect, and acceptable image quality is achievable with limited time of acoustical couplant oil application. Therefore, the rump image (**Fig. 2**A) is usually the first image collected. The rump image is collected with the transducer positioned parallel with the spine in line from the hooks to the pins, toward the dorsal aspect of the hook bone (ilium). The termination of the biceps femoris muscle is the reference point for measurement of rump fat thickness. Definition of this reference point is the most important attribute for image quality. **Fig. 2**B demonstrates the carcass anatomy in the region where the ultrasound image is being collected.

A   B

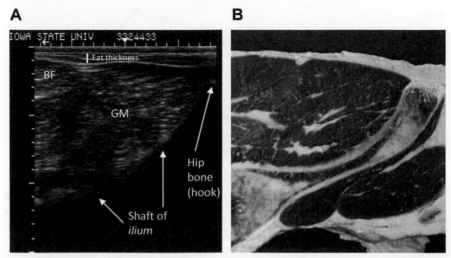

Fig. 2. (*A*) Ultrasound image collected in the rump of the animal. Hip or hook bone is an important palpation reference when collecting the image. Shaft of the ilium absorbs most of the ultrasound signal. Gluteus medius (GM) is the major muscle in this image. Termination of the biceps femoris (BF) is the reference point where the subcutaneous rump fat thickness is measured. (*B*) Picture of a carcass fabricated to demonstrate the muscle and bone structures in the rump of a beef animal. (*From* Wilson DE, Rouse GH. Beef cattle real-time ultrasound scanning guide. Iowa State University Department of Animal Science; 2002; with permission.)

2. The second image collected is a cross-sectional image between 12th and 13th thoracic vertebrae (**Fig. 3**A) and uses a standoff pad to fit the curved shape of the animal to the linear surface of the transducer. This image is used to measure 12th rib subcutaneous fat thickness at three-fourths of the lateral distance from the spine and the 12th rib longissimus cross-sectional area. **Fig. 3**B shows the carcass anatomy in the region where the ultrasound image is being collected. The most common image quality concern for this image is not being collected between the ribs, where either the 12th or the 13th rib is adversely affecting the cross-sectional area of the longissimus. **Fig. 3**C shows an extreme case of the ultrasound image being collected across the 13th vertebrae and rejected for image quality. **Fig. 3**D shows the carcass anatomy in the region where the ultrasound image is being collected. Because the ribs are not perpendicular to the ground (or the spine), finding the appropriate angle to scan between the vertebrae is the biggest challenge for the technician. If image quality is not acceptable after a short time period, typically it is a benefit to technicians to reidentify the location where they want to scan and start to collect the cross-sectional 12th rib image again.

3. Because some ultrasound technologies adjust magnification for intramuscular fat measurement and the intramuscular fat images benefit from the most time to have the acoustical couplant oil soak against the animal's skin, it is typically the last ultrasound image type collected. This longitudinal image of the longissimus is collected over the 12th to 13th vertebrae, approximately one-half to three-fourths the distance laterally across the longissimus (**Fig. 4**A). The presence of the spinalis dorsi muscle in anterior of the 12th vertebrae (**Fig. 4**B) can bias intramuscular fat interpretations, so the anterior end of the transducer may be moved laterally away from the spine to limit the presence of the spinalis dorsi in the

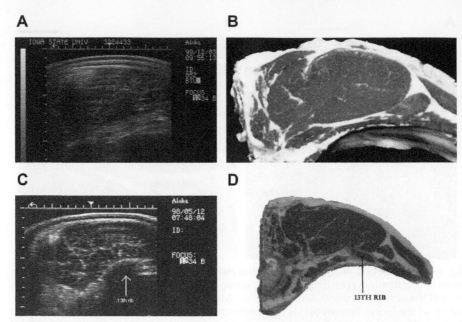

Fig. 3. (*A*) Cross-sectional ultrasound image collected between 12th and 13th thoracic vertebrae. Subcutaneous fat thickness is measured at three-quarters of the lateral distance away from the spine, and longissimus cross-sectional area is measured. (*B*) Picture of carcass at the traditional split between 12th and 13th thoracic vertebrae to separate the carcass into the front quarter and hindquarter. (*C*) Ultrasound image collected too straight up and down crossing the 13th thoracic vertebrae. (*D*) Picture of a carcass that has been cut across the 13th rib. (*From* Wilson DE, Rouse GH. Beef cattle real-time ultrasound scanning guide. Iowa State University Department of Animal Science; 2002; with permission.)

longitudinal images. **Fig. 4**C shows the carcass anatomy from the 12th thoracic vertebrae to the 10th thoracic vertebrae (anterior to the desired location for image collection). **Fig. 4**D is an ultrasound image collected too far posterior for interpretation; it shows the 13th thoracic vertebrae, then the first and second lumbar vertebrae to the left in the image (notice how lumbar vertebrae are wider and flatter topped than thoracic vertebrae). In seed stock situations the longitudinal image is used to measure intramuscular fat, but in feedlot situations the longitudinal image may also be used for subcutaneous-fat-thickness measurements to speed image collection and processing time. Because intramuscular fat is the most challenging trait to measure, 3 to 5 independent images are collected. Intramuscular fat image quality is scored as a group of 3 to 5 longitudinal images for each animal.

COMPLICATIONS AND MANAGEMENT

One of the most common complications for ultrasound measurement of carcass traits is interference picked up by the ultrasound machine. Interference renders the interpretation of intramuscular fat impossible and can influence interpretability of rump and longissimus cross-sectional images. Therefore, interference is a common reason for ultrasound image rejection by the processing laboratories. It would be expected that the breeder have a high-quality, well-grounded electrical source available for the scanning session. Additional considerations for the ultrasound technician are to (1) rearrange positions of the ultrasound machine, image-capturing computer, and

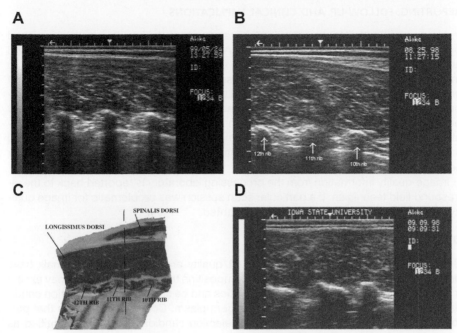

Fig. 4. (*A*) Longitudinal ultrasound image of longissimus from 13th thoracic vertebrae (*left side*) to 11th thoracic vertebrae (*right side*) for intramuscular fat measurement. Anterior of the animal is identified as being to the right of the screen because the intramuscular fat striations go ventral as they go anterior within the animal. (*B*) Longitudinal ultrasound image of longissimus collected too far anterior. Excessive spinalis dorsi between the subcutaneous fat layer and the longissimus on the right side of the screen are indicators of incorrect placement. (*C*) Picture of a carcass fabricated longitudinally to demonstrate the ultrasound image; this picture demonstrates the longissimus muscle anterior to the area of interest between the 12th and 13th thoracic vertebrae. (*D*) Longitudinal ultrasound image collected too far posterior on the animal. Left side of image shows second lumbar vertebrae, and right side of image shows 13th thoracic vertebrae; notice how thoracic vertebrae are round on the top, whereas lumbar vertebrae are wider and flatter on the top. (*From* Wilson DE, Rouse GH. Beef cattle real-time ultrasound scanning guide. Iowa State University Department of Animal Science; 2002; with permission.)

computer display; (2) consider rerouting the video and electrical cables around the ultrasound equipment; (3) externally ground the ultrasound machine; (4) be aware of electrical equipment that may be causing interference on the electric service line (eg, clippers, blowers, and so forth); and (5) use battery-powered uninterruptable power supplies/power filters to supply ultrasound imaging equipment.

From weaning until ultrasound evaluation near 1 year of age, animals need to have been managed to express a reasonable amount of their genetic potential for differences in carcass traits. Extreme nutrient restriction during the postweaning development period will limit the ability to identify genetic differences for body composition traits with ultrasound.

POSTOPERATIVE CARE

Ultrasound evaluation of body composition traits is a noninvasive procedure; animals are returned to their previous housing and feeding regimen after ultrasound scanning.

REPORTING, FOLLOW-UP, AND CLINICAL IMPLICATIONS

Images are submitted to a processing laboratory where the image quality is assessed by UGC-certified laboratory technicians. Acceptable images are interpreted, and animal identification and ultrasound body composition trait data are submitted to the beef breed association. The breed association adjusts data to their relevant end point; and raw data, adjusted data, and within-contemporary-group ratios are reported directly back to the breeder. Adjusted ultrasound trait data are used to adjust pedigree-estimated carcass trait EPD to an interim EPD until the next genetic evaluation is performed (generally 1 week to 6 months, depending on breed association) and a new carcass trait EPD for the animal becomes available. Data are used for selection and marketing purposes.

Image-quality information from the processing laboratory is reported back to the ultrasound field technician. If a particular scan session was problematic for image quality, rescanning of the animals may be warranted.

OUTCOMES

Better selection decisions for end-product quality are possible after animals have been evaluated with ultrasound for body composition traits. Some animals may exhibit a unique combination of quality characteristics and be considered as selection candidates for their unique contributions to the germplasm. Conversely, animals that performed well and seem well suited to be selection candidates may be identified as inferior for carcass quality and subsequently be culled shortly after ultrasound scanning rather than having to wait for a progeny performance evaluation.

CURRENT CONTROVERSIES

Advances in genomic technologies have introduced genomic tests that are included in carcass trait EPDs as correlated traits with nearly 1.00 heritability.[17] When producers consider that the genomic tests can influence traits beyond carcass traits, the economic considerations on whether to perform an ultrasound on candidate seed stock or perform genomic testing becomes a close decision. One consideration for producers is that they do get information about the phenotypic expression of the genetic potential under their specific management system when they evaluate candidate seed stock with ultrasound for body composition traits.

The depth of the gluteus medius muscle in the rump image has been investigated as an additional trait for retail product prediction.[7,18] Although the depth of the gluteus medius was statistically significant in predicting the retail product yield,[18] the incremental improvement was not worth the potential for less clarity and definition of the reference point when measuring rump fat thickness from the same image if widespread adoption were implemented.

FUTURE CONSIDERATIONS

There may be limitations on availability of new ultrasound equipment that has been approved by the UGC for beef cattle body composition evaluation. The current versions of ultrasound equipment used for beef cattle and lamb body composition evaluation have been very rugged and reliable. As ultrasound technology manufacturers consider phasing out that hardware, which technology will be embraced and validated through the UGC system evaluation has yet to be determined.

In the future, there may be new opportunities to use ultrasound for body composition evaluation in mature cows. Research has demonstrated high repeatability of ultrasound body composition traits in mature cows and strong relationships between ultrasound-measured body composition traits and carcass traits in mature cows.[19] There may be future opportunities to use ultrasound body composition evaluation to better characterize differences among cows for tissue depositions than the currently implemented body condition scoring system, which could lead to more precise measures of maintenance energy requirements for cows.

SUMMARY

- Ultrasound-measured body composition traits in seed stock have high genetic correlations ($\geq$0.5) with carcass traits in harvested animals.
- Beef seed stock producers have demonstrated tremendous adoption of ultrasound technology to evaluate seed stock animals for body composition traits.
- UGC certifications provide confidence to beef producers that technicians collecting and processing their ultrasound images are well qualified.
- Ultrasound body composition evaluation in beef and lambs for genetic improvement is a coordinated effort between the producer and the ultrasound technician.

REFERENCES

1. Golden BL, Garrick DJ, Newman S, et al. A framework for the next generation of EPDs. In: Proceedings Beef Improvement Federation 32nd Annual Research Symposium and Annual Meeting. Wichita (KS), July 12–15, 2000. p. 2–13.
2. USDA. United States standards for grades of carcass beef. Washington, DC: United States Department of Agriculture, Agricultural Marketing Service; 1997. Available at: http://www.ams.usda.gov/AMSv1.0/getfile?dDocName=STELDEV3002979. Accessed May 24, 2015.
3. Stoufer JR, Wallentine MV, Wellington GH, et al. Development and application of ultrasonic methods for measuring fat thickness and rib-eye area in cattle and hogs. J Anim Sci 1961;20:759–67.
4. McLaren DG, Novakofski J, Parrett DF, et al. A study of operator effects on ultrasonic measures of fat depth and longissimus muscle area in cattle, sheep, and pigs. J Anim Sci 1991;69:54–66.
5. Herring WO, Williams SE, Bertrand JK, et al. Comparison of live and carcass equations predicting percentage of cutability, retail product weight, and trimmable fat in beef cattle. J Anim Sci 1994;72:1107–18.
6. Williams RE, Bertrand JK, Williams SE, et al. Biceps femoris and rump fat as additional ultrasound measurements for predicting retail product and trimmable fat in beef carcasses. J Anim Sci 1997;75:7–13.
7. Realini CE, Williams RE, Pringle TD, et al. Gluteus medius and rump fat depths as additional live animal ultrasound measurements for predicting retail product and trimmable fat in beef carcasses. J Anim Sci 2001;79:1378–85.
8. Greiner SP, Rouse GH, Wilson DE, et al. Prediction of retail product weight and percentage using ultrasound and carcass measurements in beef cattle. J Anim Sci 2003;81:1736–42.
9. Wilson D, Rouse G, Hays C, et al. Genetic evaluation of ultrasound measures: Angus. In: Proceedings Beef Improvement Federation 31st Annual Research Symposium and Annual Meeting. Roanoke (VA), June 16–19, 1999. p. 197–8.
10. MacNeil MD, Northcutt SL. National cattle evaluation system for combined analysis of carcass characteristics and indicator traits recorded by using ultrasound in Angus cattle. J Anim Sci 2008;86:2518–24.

11. American Angus Association. American Angus Association spring 2001 sire evaluation edition. St. Joseph (MO): Angus Journal, Angus Productions, Inc; 2001.

12. American Angus Association. American Angus Association spring 2015 sire evaluation edition. St. Joseph (MO): Angus Journal, Angus Productions, Inc; 2015. Available at: http://www.angus.org/Nce/Carcass.aspx. Accessed May 17, 2015.

13. Brethour JR. Using serial ultrasound measures to generate models of marbling and backfat thickness changes in feedlot cattle. J Anim Sci 2000;78:2055–61.

14. Wall PB, Rouse GH, Wilson DE, et al. Use of ultrasound to predict body composition changes in steers at 100 and 65 days before slaughter. J Anim Sci 2004;82:1621–9.

15. Emenheiser JC, Greiner SP, Lewis RM, et al. Validation of live animal ultrasonic measurements of body composition in market lambs. J Anim Sci 2010;88:2932–9.

16. Notter D. NSIP EBV notebook. Harlan (IA): National Sheep Improvement Program; 2011. Available at: http://nsip.org/wp-content/uploads/2015/03/NSIP-EBV-Descriptions-FINAL-1.16.15.pdf. Accessed May 26, 2015.

17. MacNeil MD, Nkrumah JD, Woodward BW, et al. Genetic evaluation of Angus cattle for carcass marbling using ultrasound and genomic indicators. J Anim Sci 2010;88:517–22.

18. Tait RG Jr, Wilson DE, Rouse GH. Prediction of retail product and trimmable fat yields from the four primal cuts in beef cattle using ultrasound or carcass data. J Anim Sci 2005;83:1353–60.

19. Emenheiser JC, Tait RG Jr, Shackelford SD, et al. Use of ultrasound scanning and body condition score to evaluate composition traits in mature beef cows. J Anim Sci 2014;92:3868–77.

Index

Note: Page numbers of article titles are in **boldface** type.

A

Moving?

Make sure your subscription moves with you!

To notify us of your new address, find your **Clinics Account Number** (located on your mailing label above your name), and contact customer service at:

Email: journalscustomerservice-usa@elsevier.com

800-654-2452 (subscribers in the U.S. & Canada)
314-447-8871 (subscribers outside of the U.S. & Canada)

Fax number: 314-447-8029

Elsevier Health Sciences Division
Subscription Customer Service
3251 Riverport Lane
Maryland Heights, MO 63043

*To ensure uninterrupted delivery of your subscription, please notify us at least 4 weeks in advance of move.

Printed and bound by CPI Group (UK) Ltd, Croydon, CR0 4YY

07/10/2024

01040499-0009